"Your child overeats. Put down the idea that now your job is to be the diet police. This problem is way more important—and way more hopeful—than that. You and your child have a chance to learn how the mind and body work. This wise book will help you and your child learn to see thoughts and feelings for what they really are, making it more possible for your child or teen to make mindful choices, to build healthy habits, and to live a healthy, values-based life without the burden of shame and self-criticism. Turn this problem into the opportunity that it is. This wonderful book will show you how."

—STEVEN C. HAYES, PhD, professor, University of Nevada, codeveloper of Acceptance and Commitment Therapy and author of *Get Out of Your Mind and Into Your Life*

"*Free Your Child from Overeating* helps parents work with their children on health and wellness without stress and worry. This book gives parents and teens all the tools they will need to succeed."

—MARCI G. FOX, PhD, licensed psychologist and coauthor of *Think Confident, Be Confident for Teens*

"This handbook provides priceless strategies to help parents and their children raise self-esteem, overcome cravings, and strengthen communication. To achieve lasting success, parents must model healthy, active behavior for their children to emulate. This book will guide parents, step-by-step, one bite at a time."

—CORBIN BILLINGS, director of the documentary *Bite Size*

"A tour de force, Dr. Michelle Maidenberg's *Free Your Child from Overeating* is complete, inspiring, and pragmatic. Speaking with a voice that's both personal and professional, Dr. Maidenberg gives parents and their children the impossible—a way to actually create a space between desire and action, between wanting food and actually eating it, between an impulse and the self-contempt many feel after binging or simply eating when not hungry."

—MARK R. BANSCHICK, MD, author of *The Intelligent Divorce*

"Getting clear guidance on nutrition and health can be an incredibly frustrating endeavor. Dr. Michelle Maidenberg has the answer! Parents of children who overeat will find a wealth of helpful resources, thought-provoking exercises, and sound advice in this book."

—CRAIG HAEN, PhD, psychotherapist and author of *Engaging Boys in Treatment: Creative Approaches to the Therapy Process*

"Dr. Maidenberg's framework, grounded in mindfulness and acceptance and commitment therapy, weaves empathy, unconditional acceptance, and care throughout each activity in this book. From 'stinking thinking' to 'the cupcake conundrum,' Dr. Maidenberg has created a brilliant guide to help parents and children lead healthier lives."

—SUSAN CIARDIELLO, PhD, LCSW, psychotherapist and ADHD coach, author of *ACTivities for Group Work with School-Age Children* and *ACTivities for Group Work with Adolescents*

"*Free Your Child from Overeating* utilizes a step-by-step, practical, and innovative approach and teaches parents (and others caring for kids such as nutritionists and pediatricians) how to empower kids and teens to take responsibility for their health in a proactive and highly effective manner."

—ANN GOELITZ, PhD, LCSW-R, psychotherapist and author of *From Trauma to Healing: A Social Worker's Guide to Working with Survivors*

"This is an excellent, clearly written, easily understood, and helpful book that presents solutions to the serious problem of overweight children. It helps parents who often feel powerless about helping their child."

—ROBERT SCHACHTER, EdD, assistant clinical professor, department of psychiatry, Icahn School of Medicine at Mount Sinai

"Using a family-based approach, Dr. Maidenberg brilliantly provides a series of user-friendly strategies for implementing behavior change. This book focuses on nutrition habits and behaviors, rather than weight, and provides the missing link for success in pediatric weight management. It is a must-read for any family looking to introduce more mindfulness around eating."

—WENDY STERLING, MS, RD, CSSD, sports nutritionist, eating disorder expert, and former nutritionist for the New York Jets

"As a clinician, I often see the serious effects of overeating. Dr. Maidenberg's book is a necessary primer for all parents to start to learn very practical strategies that can set the right tone for helping their kids and teens from the beginning. *Free Your Child from Overeating* is thoughtful, thorough, practical, and scholarly."

—JENNIE J. KRAMER, MSW, LCSW, founder and executive director of Metro Behavioral Health Associates Eating Disorder Treatment Centers and coauthor of *Overcoming Binge Eating for Dummies*

"Dr. Michelle Maidenberg's solid, well-researched, and exceedingly practical handbook on family wellness—body, mind, and spirit—reads like a breath of fresh air. *Free Your Child from Overeating* helps families avoid 'magic bullet' mantras and head simply and easily toward a legacy of health."

—BRENDA WOLLENBERG, BSW, RHN, author of *Overweight Kids in a Toothpick World* and founder of In Balance Wellness and Weight Release Programs

FREE YOUR CHILD from OVEREATING

A Handbook for Helping Kids and Teens

 53 Mind-Body Strategies for Lifelong Health

MICHELLE P. MAIDENBERG,

PhD, MPH, LCSW-R

THE EXPERIMENT

NEW YORK

The Experiment, LLC
220 East 23rd Street, Suite 301
New York, NY 10010-4674
www.theexperimentpublishing.com

This book contains the opinions and ideas of its author. It is intended to provide helpful and informative material on the subjects addressed in the book. It is sold with the understanding that the author and publisher are not engaged in rendering medical, health, or any other kind of personal professional services in the book. The author and publisher specifically disclaim all responsibility for any liability, loss, or risk—personal or otherwise—that is incurred as a consequence, directly or indirectly, of the use and application of any of the contents of this book.

Many of the designations used by manufacturers and sellers to distinguish their products are claimed as trademarks. Where those designations appear in this book and The Experiment was aware of a trademark claim, the designations have been capitalized.

The Experiment's books are available at special discounts when purchased in bulk for premiums and sales promotions as well as for fund-raising or educational use. For details, contact us at info@theexperimentpublishing.com.

Library of Congress Cataloging-in-Publication Data

Names: Maidenberg, Michelle, author.
Title: Free your child from overeating : a handbook for helping kids and
  teens / Michelle Maidenberg.
Description: New York : The Experiment, [2016] | Includes bibliographical
  references and index.
Identifiers: LCCN 2015006022| ISBN 9781615192700 (pbk.) | ISBN 9781615192717
  (ebook)
Subjects: LCSH: Eating disorders in children--Treatment. | Acceptance and
  commitment therapy.
Classification: LCC RJ506.E18 M33 2015 | DDC 618.92/8526--dc23
LC record available at http://lccn.loc.gov/2015006022

ISBN 978-1-61519-270-0
Ebook ISBN 978-1-61519-271-7

Cover design by Sarah Smith
Text design by Pauline Neuwirth
Author photo by Matt Carr

Manufactured in the United States of America
Distributed by Workman Publishing Company, Inc.
Distributed simultaneously in Canada by Thomas Allen & Son Ltd.

First printing March 2016
10 9 8 7 6 5 4 3 2 1

To Eric, my beloved husband,
whose support is unconditional and fierce

CONTENTS

INTRODUCTION

CHILDHOOD AND TEEN OBESITY has grown to epidemic proportions in the United States. The numbers are stark and speak for themselves. As of 2010, more than one-third of the children and adolescents in this country were overweight or obese. The Centers for Disease Control and Prevention, the United States National Center for Health Statistics, and the *Journal of the American Medical Association* have confirmed that obesity has more than doubled in children and tripled in adolescents in the past thirty years.

The percentage of children six to eleven years of age in the United States who were obese increased from 7 percent in 1980 to nearly 18 percent in 2010. Similarly, the percentage of adolescents ages twelve to nineteen who were obese increased from 5 percent to 18 percent over the same period. In 2011 to 2014, 8.9 percent of two- to five-year-olds were obese compared with 17.5 percent of six- to eleven-year-olds and 20.5 percent of twelve- to nineteen-year-olds. Although the prevalence rates of youth obesity did not change in studies from 2003 to 2004 and 2013 to 2014, there has not been any decrease in them, either, and the rates remain staggering.[1]

There are serious and immediate physical and psychological effects to being overweight and obese, such as prediabetes, bone and joint problems, social issues, and poor self-confidence, as well as long-term risks to our children. Heart disease, stroke, poor self-image/identity, and depression are some of the many problems that can persist from childhood through adulthood due to weight and health issues. The medical and economic toll of this problem remains huge, as well. It is estimated that the obesity epidemic carries a $117 billion medical price tag.[2]

What remains confusing is that, although there is a plethora of resources available—from school health classes to online sources, to mainstream

books on integrating healthy eating and effective exercise regimens—
obesity is still a growing trend. Why are we still experiencing a dispropor-
tionate number of kids and teens who are overweight and obese?

WHAT HAVE WE TRIED?

Given the gravity of this issue, government agencies, institutions, and
individuals are working diligently to identify best practices to alleviate
the problem. We are all concerned about the health and wellness of our
children and future generations and eagerly seek strategies that will
work.

What have we tried? We've increased general awareness and the availability of resources regarding nutrition and exercise standards for people
of all ages. However, just because the information is out there doesn't
mean that people are using it or putting it into practice. Some have
adopted admirable methods of educating children and parents about the
risks of being overweight and obese, as well as ways to adopt better habits
with respect to proper nutrition and exercise.

The fact is, you as a parent must understand what you've been taught,
which is often challenging because of the confusing and opposing advice
that's offered. You also have to interpret it for the situations you and your
child face, and then communicate it effectively to your child. Furthermore,
you are expected to serve as a role model for your child at the same time
that you are enforcing certain strategies and standards at home, a two-
pronged task that is difficult but critical to long-term success for your
child and family.

Traditionally, you have had to carry out all of these tasks alone. There
are a limited number of formalized programs and support groups for kids
and teens. *Free Your Child from Overeating* is a comprehensive handbook
that can help. This mind-body approach deals with all facets of the overeating and obesity issue. New research has found mind-body approaches
to be significantly effective in long-term youth health outcomes.[3] It is
important to take into consideration the biological, social, political, and
economic complexities of a public health issue such as obesity. However,
a key component has not been adequately addressed—the psychological
barriers to dealing with this disease. In order to achieve fundamental
long-term change, we must address these psychological barriers.

Why is it critical to understand the psychological component? Not
only do kids and teens have to face normal physical and emotional

changes, but in our ever-developing, tech-focused world, they now have new pressures to deal with that never existed before. The constant barrage of media and social messages about how they "should" look, feel, and behave enters their consciousness 24/7. Kids and teens are constantly inundated with ideas about what it means to be happy, healthy, and successful. Now, as a parent, you are not only responsible for helping them navigate the expected ups and downs of being a teen; you must also help them deal with an ever-changing kaleidoscope of challenges that weren't necessarily part of your own experience.

Kids and teens don't choose to be overweight. Undoubtedly, if they could control it, wouldn't they? Why would they choose to endure the negative consequences of being overweight? We also now know that food can be addictive. For children especially, the neurochemical reward center in the brain can override "willpower" and overwhelm the biological signals that control hunger. Thus, they truly cannot help overeating. We need to provide kids and teens with resources and guidance to help them with this challenge.

The strategies in this book will teach you and your child concrete skills for working through psychological barriers in an engaging, easy-to-understand way. It will provide you with ways to evaluate your child's understanding and give clear guidance on how to convey and reinforce the information with your child. The strategies are not one-size-fits-all; they focus on the unique needs of kids and teens and their families and assist with sustaining change over time.

TRANSFORMING THE LIVES OF KIDS AND TEENS

If you are the parent of an overweight or obese child or teen, you are probably overwhelmed with the challenge of watching your child struggle. You probably tried cutting back on sweets or seeing a nutritionist for a diet plan, but nothing has worked. Even if it has, the results were likely temporary and not sustainable. At times you feel frustrated and angry at yourself and your child, and mostly you worry about this issue getting out of control and its long-term negative effects. You accept that it is your responsibility to teach your children about healthy living and maintaining a reasonable weight. How are you going to do it? Likely no one ever taught you, and you are not sure where to start or how to go about it.

It's not your or your child's fault; you and your child likely have been taught treatment approaches that only scratch the surface and do not create true behavioral change. Whenever I speak on this topic, I ask the audience who among them has dieted and lost weight in their lifetime, and all hands go up. However, when I ask the same group whether they were able to maintain their weight loss, few hands get raised.

Knowing how to sustain long-term change is what is missing for most kids and teens. This book addresses what factors get in your child's way and teaches you how to work through them together. *Free Your Child from Overeating* helps you learn how to work with your child to identify and define your child's core values, while at the same time working on behavior, so that change is made at the core and not just peripherally.

WHY I CAN HELP

My personal journey is relevant in explaining why I feel so compelled to work with others on lifelong health and wellness. I am a person who practices what she preaches, and I know my methods work because I practice them every day, both personally and professionally.

One of the reasons I'm so passionate about my work is my own history with health and weight challenges. Throughout my formative years, a number of circumstances put me in the position of being vulnerable to overeating. Food was reliable and consistent. It was also something I could control. It is not very surprising at all that I found comfort in food.

During my preteens and teens, I was tall but overweight. The last straw came when I gained 15 to 20 pounds during my first year of college. I came home feeling even more overweight and frustrated than before. But this time I decided, that was it. I wanted to make a change to be healthier and to feel better about myself. I adopted a healthier diet, integrated a consistent exercise regimen into my life, and eventually became an aerobics instructor to make some extra money while attending college and graduate school. I lost approximately 40 pounds and kept it off for all these years (twenty-seven in total!), excluding the time during my four pregnancies.

During each of my pregnancies, I gained 75 pounds, for a total of 300 pounds. It was a substantial amount of weight, but my body did what it did, even with exercising until the day I gave birth and eating relatively healthily. After each birth, I worked diligently to get back into shape and lose the weight I'd gained. Each birth brought its own challenges, but I was successfully able to reach the goal of losing the weight I'd gained.

In my practice and in my life I have seen people suffer physically and psychologically as a result of overeating. I meet many individuals who want to make a positive change but simply do not know how to connect their minds to their actions. Fundamental change only comes when people are able to link what they think and feel to the way they behave and live according to their values.

The following skills have become a habitual, philosophical, and behavioral shift for me. I predict, plan, put into action, and practice (the 4Ps, the model the book is based on) things that will help me face challenges. I am aware of my patterns of thinking, feeling, and behaving relative to eating. I don't deny my impulses, hide from them, or avoid them. I lean into my feelings, observe them, and revel at my humanness while I stay on my toes and remind myself how important it is for me to remain healthy and live a meaningful life. I continually practice these skills, and they are now fully incorporated into the way I function.

Most books about diet on the market are written by physicians, nutritionists, or behavioral coaches who use a medical model to provide nutritional tips and exercise guidelines. Too often they are geared solely toward physiological factors alone, with limited or no inclusion of the psychological and emotional factors that affect weight-loss progress. My knowledge and expertise in human behavior and cognitive development lend to a unique approach in this book.

I have advanced training in Structural Family Therapy, Cognitive-Behavioral Therapy (CBT), Acceptance and Commitment Therapy (ACT), and Eye Movement Desensitization Reprocessing (EMDR). I see individual clients in my practice, have run groups for weight loss and weight management, and have developed and supervise the CBT weight-loss and weight-management program at Camp Shane (for children and teens) and Shane Diet and Fitness Resorts (for young adults and adults). I also teach CBT and human behavior at New York University in the school's graduate social work program.

I have had the privilege of conducting focus groups with parents, kids, and teens at the Boys & Girls Clubs of Mount Vernon, New York. There, parents, kids, and teens talked candidly about their personal experiences with weight and health issues at home, in school, and within their families. I have also conducted additional focus groups with select groups of kids and teens, parents, physicians, nutritionists, nurse practitioners, psychotherapists, health coaches, and trainers. I consciously chose to study a wide range of diverse populations by using a structured questionnaire with all these groups to ensure that I addressed the needs of most kids and teens.

I have attempted to convey my resulting insights in a way that's easily understood and applied. This book represents an exciting opportunity for me to help you in a meaningful and fundamental way. I am honored to be able to share all that I have learned with you.

WHO THIS BOOK IS FOR

This book was written for parents, to enable you to learn and work conjointly with your ten- to eighteen-year-old child. The strategies outlined provide flexibility, depending on how old your child is, how open your child is to this process, and how comfortable with and willing your child is to share and interact with you about health challenges. You and your child will work collaboratively to learn the strategies and complete the exercises I offer. Kids and teens can also choose to work more independently, or they can elect to work with other individuals who can support them through the process.

It is understandable that every child will approach the matters this book addresses at different levels of readiness and desire to change behaviors. You, the parent, will learn precepts from motivational interviewing (MI), an evidence-based counseling approach, in order to enhance your child's engagement in this process. If your child is putting up resistance from the outset, reading up on these skills may help you. These skills include setting small, specific, and realistic goals, asking open-ended questions, providing positive and helpful feedback, engaging in reflective or "active" listening, and doing so in a nonjudgmental and nonconfrontational manner.[4] The focus is on building confidence, increasing motivation, and creating behavioral change. Techniques to help you help your child to increase readiness and desire for change will be outlined throughout this book.

This book can also assist pediatricians, adolescent-medicine physicians, internists, endocrinologists, nutritionists, health coaches, advocates for children's health, etc., who would benefit from learning these skills and/or who want to work directly with their patients/clients in an engaging and helpful way.

This book is a good supplement to any program that advocates healthful eating and exercise practices. Incorporating a comprehensive approach is useful and highly effective. I recommend that you and your child get educated on nutrition and healthy physical-activity practices. Also, if there is any underlying psychological or social challenge, it should be addressed first, or it might get in the way and block your child from learning and integrating the strategies. An example of this is if your child has social anxiety and subconsciously uses weight gain as a means to avoid social interactions.

Be aware of eating patterns and beliefs that may indicate an eating disorder.[5] Some signs to look out for are: (1) skipping meals or making excuses for not eating, (2) hyper-focusing on food and eating, (3) adopting an overly restrictive diet, (4) dread and embarrassment about eating in public, (5) social isolation or withdrawing from social activities, (6) persistent worry or complaining about being overweight, (7) frequently checking the mirror for perceived flaws or talking about perceived flaws, (8) repeatedly and compulsively eating large amounts of food, (9) excessive use of dietary supplements, laxatives, or herbal products for weight loss, (10) excessive exercising, (11) inducing vomiting, and (12) expressing depression, disgust, shame, or guilt about eating habits. If your child has an eating disorder, it's best to seek professional help and approach the skills I outline following recovery or when it is deemed therapeutically appropriate.

WHAT MAKES THIS BOOK UNIQUE

Presently, many books focus on nutrition, exercise, or on developing healthy habits. This book deals with all three topics and how they are intertwined while simultaneously looking at the world we live in and how it affects our children. Additionally, I tackle the issues facing every parent of a child and teen: the best ways to communicate and collaborate with your child; how to address biological, psychological, and social development; how to deal with siblings; and what to do when you're at your wits' end. I also discuss children's social lives, media influences, the effects of today's technology, and what it means to live healthfully.

I take great care to make sure the emphasis is on making empowering changes that are guided by your child's values rather than on getting rid of negative traits or characteristics, which would convey that parts of your child are "bad" or "unworthy." The book utilizes the 4Ps model—predict, plan, put into action, and practice—which further emphasizes making change in a lasting way.

My book stresses acceptance and appreciation—for parents, children, and families. Through encouragement, support, and care, you *can* teach your child to make mindful choices that work.

Each chapter of *Free Your Child from Overeating* has select strategies with pertinent information, tips, and exercises that reinforce the skills taught in the chapter. The exercises are for you to share with your child. Your child can write in the book in the spaces provided where applicable. Or you may want to purchase a notebook for your child to write down responses, keep track of the exercises completed, and explore thoughts and feelings more deeply. For tech-savvy kids and teens, they can also use their computer or smartphone to keep track of their goals and other tips they may want to refer to on a daily basis.

The chapters contain quotations from kids and parents I have interviewed throughout my research, as well as a section called "Check Your Baggage," which encourages you as a parent to check in with yourself regarding any thoughts and feelings that may have been evoked throughout your learning and conveying of the strategies, and how those may directly impact interaction with your child. Following this there is a brief "Review" section. The review sections are general but include bulleted lists addressed to parents or kids and teens.

At the end of each chapter is a reference to a guided mindfulness-based exercise (collected at the end of the book with instructions for accessing online audio files) that further reinforces the skills presented. The purpose of the mindfulness-based exercise is to teach parents and children to slow down, to be present and in the moment, to integrate the skills being taught, and to increase their mind and body awareness. Mindfulness has been proven to facilitate clarity in focusing and processing, to boost working memory, to enable more cognitive flexibility and less emotional reactivity, and to work as an effective stress reducer. This will be explored in depth in the opening chapter.

WHY LEARNING THESE SKILLS IS IMPORTANT

This book is applicable to all families. Although its primary audience is families in which overeating and weight pose challenges, it is also a manual for all families to learn to communicate about the importance of healthy living. Learning about the way the mind functions, the process of accepting ourselves for who we are, and working toward understanding our health values are skills that are of use to everyone. This work fosters independent thinking and the ability to problem solve. It is an empowering approach that suggests that meaningful behavioral change can happen with practice, effort, and ingenuity.

With regard to eating and weight, people are always maturing, developing, and growing. As we age, our metabolism changes, and our weight tends to fluctuate. By acquiring communication skills, problem-solving abilities, and coping skills early on, we can help ourselves and our kids experience positive personal growth.

Even though a child may develop without weight or health issues, as people evolve and mature, eating and exercise eventually become something we all need to manage at some point. Understanding how we think, feel, and behave in regard to our eating and health in general are strategies from which we can all benefit.

These strategies and skills are relevant and user-friendly for any individual or family. They can be easily taught, reviewed, reinforced, and reintroduced at any point in time.

ON YOUR WAY

You took the first step and picked up this book! This promises to be an eye-opening exploration and one well worth embarking on. Taking inventory and truly accepting who you and your child are by working with your and your child's full array of thoughts, feelings, and behaviors will fundamentally promote long-term changes, and not just a temporary shift like you may have experienced in the past. I thank you for having the courage and willingness to discuss a topic that often evokes intense feelings, and for the care you are demonstrating to your child by guiding them through this process. And thank you for attempting to open up lines of communication and connection with your child.

Think about how many times you've tried to make healthy changes (just like everyone else—it's not just you!). How much money, time, and energy have you spent on projects that just served as a Band-Aid? This time will be different for you and your family. Don't you want you and your child to be the ones to raise your hands when I ask if you have maintained healthful eating and exercise behaviors for the long term? I want so much for that to be you, too. This book is written with warmth, care, and support for you and your family. I truly appreciate your taking this journey.

Being Present

Every night after dinner, I find that I crave dessert. I wish it were the healthy kind. Sometimes I'm able to control it, and sometimes I'm not. When I'm not, I'm left feeling defeated and very shameful. I feel so weak and frustrated that I even have to deal with this.

—MATTHEW, AGE 18

I try so hard to control myself when I'm at sweet sixteens. There's so much amazing food. It overwhelms me, and I give in. I wish these thoughts would just go away. —SARA, AGE 16

THE COMEDIAN EMO PHILIPS SAID, "I used to think my mind was the most important organ. Then I noticed what organ was telling me that." Psychologist Steven Hayes, one of the creators of Acceptance and Commitment Therapy (ACT), once referenced this quotation in an article. Hayes went on to say, "The human mind is arrogant beyond belief. Because our minds can talk about anything, this organ between our ears thinks it knows everything. Our logical, analytical, predictive, problem-solving mind knows how to live, knows how to love, and knows how to be at peace. Not."[6]

Our minds are constantly buzzing and playing games—and seemingly have minds of their own. This often puts us in a loop of struggling with our thoughts, while having thoughts about our thoughts (not to mention feelings about our feelings!). Why does this matter? Because our thoughts have a direct impact on our eating and exercise behaviors.

Traditionally, you learn that if you eat well and exercise, you'll be healthy. Even though it seems simple, many kids and teens (and adults, too!) have trouble sticking to the simple A+B = C formula. The trouble is, a formula does not take our thinking and emotions into account. Being aware of your and your child's thoughts and feelings and how they impact eating and exercise behaviors opens up the possibility of an ongoing practice of curiosity, self-awareness, and committed action toward health. Then, the equation results in improved health. This is a mind-body approach for kids and teens that will eventually affect all aspects of their lives. The beauty is that they do not need to go outside of themselves to find the answer; it is already living within them.

Integrating mindful awareness creates space for you and your child to pay attention to the thoughts and feelings that regularly impact behavior. With awareness, you and your child get to decide which behaviors are in line with your values and goals. By working collaboratively, you can make changes that benefit both of you over the long term.

The concepts and exercises in this book are grounded in Cognitive-Behavioral Therapy (CBT), Acceptance and Commitment Therapy (ACT), and mindfulness practice. CBT has been around for more than fifty years, and mindfulness has been practiced for millennia by Buddhists and those who have embraced other Eastern philosophies; however, it is only within the past twenty years (ACT was created in the late eighties) that these methods have been applied, researched, and studied in the context of weight loss and weight management.

Using these evidenced-based methods allows for sustained and incremental change at one's core, rather than change that is fleeting, which often happens with quick-fix fad diets and exercise regimens. The transformation starts with helping your child connect to values as they relate to health (this will be further explored in Chapter 2) and leads to enhanced self-awareness, self-acceptance, self-confidence, self-love, and an all-around better quality of life in body and mind. These are the ultimate goals that you undoubtedly desire for your child.

At the end of each chapter, a section called "Check Your Baggage" encourages you to check in and notice your own thoughts and feelings that may come up during the process—and that in turn may impact your child. Each chapter also concludes with a "Review" checklist of the skills discussed and a reference to a mindfulness exercise.

MIND BUZZ

Understand How the Mind Works

Millions of thoughts, both positive and negative, pass through our minds all day long. That's part of what makes us human. On the one hand, it's amazing and wondrous, but if we're trying to get through to our kids, it can be the most frustrating thing in the world to try to break through the constant buzz of ideas and information running through their heads day and night. If we attempt to have a conversation about *anything* other than technology, sports, school, music, fashion, or friendships, they're probably not all that interested. And if we want to talk to them about something serious, forget it!

Like many adults, kids and teens want to control their thoughts because they affect how they feel. You may be familiar with beating yourself up for having uncomfortable thoughts, trying desperately to avoid them, and attempting in many ways to rid yourself of them. Kids and teens struggle with the same battle.

At times, we all struggle with "crazy," "irrational," and "unwanted" thoughts we wish we could control or never have to begin with. And what's even more uncomfortable is that those very thoughts often lead to negative feelings. Who wants to admit to them? Who wants to carry them around? Across the board, everyone prefers to hold on to positive thoughts and avoid negative ones.

For example, it's just after dinner and your daughter is eyeing the left-over snack her brother left on the counter after emptying out his backpack. She knows she just ate and thinks, "I really want those pretzels. What's the big deal? I won't have a snack tomorrow." These thoughts are followed by, "Who are you kidding? You'll have that and more snacks tomorrow. You won't be able to resist."

Feelings of exasperation and hopelessness then follow a string of other thoughts: "I'm such a loser, why can't I get this right, why can't my mind just be quiet!" At this point the hopelessness intensifies even more, and she says, "At least I'll feel better if I eat them." She eats the pretzels and is left feeling ashamed, sad, and helpless.

Wouldn't it be nice if your child could turn feelings on and off like a light switch? Then, she could turn on the ones she wants to hold on to because they're comfortable and make her feel good, and turn off the ones that make her disappointed, frustrated, or angry. In reality, kids and teens find themselves avoiding uncomfortable feelings by distracting themselves with various activities or by quickly giving in to the thoughts to quiet down the chatter. Avoidance and surrender strategies help in the short term but in the long run leave kids with even more intensely uncomfortable feelings about their circumstances and selves. Surrendering also perpetuates the negative self-talk, because the circumstances seem grimmer and the negative thoughts are validated.

Trying to make thoughts go away is exhausting and takes up a lot of brain space. It also doesn't work, no matter how hard we try.

EXERCISE: Accepting, Not Controlling, Thoughts

Try this exercise with your child. Ask her to pick a number from one to five. Then ask her to repeat that number five times. Instruct her that she has three minutes to forget the number and that she should try as hard as she can to forget it. Let her know she can pull out all the stops and has free rein to implement any and all strategies that she would like to use to accomplish this. Give her three minutes to mull it over.

Following the three minutes, ask her if she was successful at forgetting the number. The following day, ask her if she still remembers the number. You'll both have a good laugh! The number is there to stay. She'll quickly see how, as much as she would like to, her thoughts are her thoughts, and she can't control them.

An important step both you and your child must take is to accept that she can't control her thoughts, feelings, or bodily sensations. But she *can* control her behavior and the actions she chooses to take.

STRATEGY 2

MIND GAMES

Listen to the Messages Your Mind Conveys

It's only natural to play mind games with ourselves to rationalize getting what we want. Your child may have an initial thought or feeling about food; then, he layers it with judgment, criticism, evaluation, analyzing, and planning. He ends up with thoughts about his thoughts, feelings about his feelings, or criticisms about them. For example, a teenager struggling with his weight and trying to make changes might think, "Okay, I just ate dinner and dessert. I feel full, but I still want seconds on the dessert."

13

Then, he considers the options: "I know I just ate dinner, but I still want it," or, "Even though I'm full, there's still more room for a bit more," or, "Just this one time. I deserve it, since I had a really hard day at school." He may also judge his thoughts: "Why can't I just control myself?" "Why do I have to think that it is just one time?" "Why can't I realize that it is not just one more time? It's all the time!" And the negative thoughts continue:

"I'm so frustrated at myself for having these thoughts."

"I'm such an idiot for having them and giving in to them."

"I have no control over myself."

"I'll never be able to do this."

"What's the point?"

This string of thoughts about thoughts and feelings about feelings may lead him to feel ashamed, guilty, and ineffective. That might lead him to act impulsively—for example, by taking seconds on dessert even though it goes against his plan. He might overlook that he had these thoughts and feelings at all, which wouldn't leave any room for contemplation, processing, problem solving, and acting mindfully with self-awareness.

Kids and teens are notoriously impulsive, and when your child struggles to make changes to his eating and exercise behavior, the mind plays an important, if not *the* most important, role. Without ever having learned what to do in the face of temptation, kids and teens may not give themselves the time to mull over their thoughts about eating because they are reacting to them so quickly. Instead, as in the example mentioned, they often try to rid themselves of their uncomfortable thoughts, either consciously or subconsciously, by either avoiding them or impulsively acting on them. And even if they are aware of those thoughts and take time to evaluate them, they might still decide they want to eat seconds on dessert, anyway—because "it tastes good" and they "must have it."

Whatever the case, as a parent encouraging a child, it's key to remember that thoughts may shift, may not be rational at times, and may change based on circumstances. No matter how ingrained your child's eating habits are, change can still happen. All of us can learn to slow down and act mindfully, gain more awareness about ourselves, and learn ways that we can cope with situations in a manner that reflects our goals and values.

Although your child can't control his thoughts, the good news is that he can make an effort to observe them, understand them, evaluate them, and make decisions based on what leads him in the direction of his values. As you help him learn how to problem solve through these kinds of challenges, you may become better at it, as well. Then, together, your

14

family can decide if your thoughts—and, more important, the actions they lead to—are in line with how you want to live your lives and make changes if necessary.

Tell your child, "You have more control than you realize!" Your mind often trips you up and puts you in a position of doubting yourself, rationalizing your behavior, and convincing you of what you *should* be doing. But you *still* get to decide! If you learn more about how your mind works and retrain yourself to approach your thoughts with curiosity, flexibility, and self-compassion, it no longer has to be this way. *It's important to remember that the thing that gets between you and your values is you.*

Further share with him the need to be aware of the games our minds all play, which lead to thoughts about thoughts and to feelings about feelings. Being more aware also helps stop the negative sentiments that chip away at his self-worth and self-compassion. A child is less likely to make changes if he doesn't believe in himself or have the confidence to accomplish his goals and act in accordance with his value of health.

EXERCISE: Tracking Mind Games

Ask your child to track his thoughts for two days and identify the following "layers" of his thoughts when he is confronted with a challenging situation. They are bound to come up! He should identify the circumstance, what his basic thought is, what thought follows, how he feels about the thought, how he feels about the feeling, how else he can see the situation and what potential options are available to him, and what his mind is telling him to do. Here's an example he can follow:

CIRCUMSTANCE: I am at my cousin's house, and she offers me a chocolate bar.

BASIC THOUGHT: "I have to have it; it's being offered to me."

THOUGHT THAT FOLLOWS: "I wish I didn't have this thought and could just say no. There's something seriously wrong with me."

FEELING ABOUT THE THOUGHT: Frustrated, disappointed, and angered

FEELING ABOUT THE FEELING: Sad and hopeless

HOW ELSE YOU CAN SEE THE SITUATION AND WHAT OPTIONS ARE AVAILABLE: (a) I can have the chocolate bar and say nothing, (b) not have it and say something, or (c) have some of it and say something.

WHAT YOUR MIND IS TELLING YOU TO DO: To eat the candy bar and not say anything.

What if he were to gently and compassionately be open to his thoughts and feelings, rather than trying to avoid or get rid of them? He could accept that in general it's hard for him to assert himself because of his perception that, in this case, he'll offend and hurt his cousin.

He would also need to consider that when he wants something to eat, it is hard for him to sit with the frustration, so he usually just gives in to his craving. If he chooses to take action based on his values, he might notice that he is not hungry and this is simply a craving, assert himself respectfully (while still having the fear), and sit with the frustration of not having the chocolate. Going through this process, he would be exercising assertiveness skills, frustration tolerance, and problem-solving skills. If he impulsively just gives in to the craving, he would deprive himself of all this growth and learning.

STRATEGY 3

THOUGHTS HAVE A MIND OF THEIR OWN

Understand Thought Patterns

Without a doubt, *thoughts have a mind of their own.* They run wild, and your child may automatically and wholeheartedly treat her thoughts as facts. Sometimes she may even assume that there is only one way to understand them, which might lead her to think there's only one way to handle a situation. Therefore, your child's behavior reflects the "facts" she considers her thoughts to be. Many adults still navigate the world according to this simplistic understanding of thoughts, so it's likely that your child has learned over time to see things through a similar black-and-white lens.

It's important to consider how your thoughts and feelings align or conflict with your health values and goals, even before you bring your child into this process. I encourage you to challenge and investigate your own thinking, so you can understand any preexisting patterns in your thinking, what impacts your thinking, and your usual range of feelings so that you will be able to help your child do the same.

By looking at yourself and your thoughts with fresh eyes, you will become curious and begin to question, consider, and make more mindful decisions over time and with practice. And by reframing your own thought processes and retraining your brain, you can successfully model the kind of problem solving and action that is the basis for success and lifelong weight management for yourself and your children.

EXERCISE: Thoughts Are Not Facts

As a family, you have an opportunity to delve into your minds, learn more about how you feel based on your thoughts, consider why you think and feel a certain way, assess what options you have, and open yourself to alternative ways of behaving.

First practice asking yourself these questions, then ask your child. These questions can lead to rich discussion so that you are jointly learning more about your thoughts and feelings.

- Where do your thoughts generally lead?
- What typically brings on the thoughts?
- Do these tend to be new or older thoughts? (Consistent, predictable thoughts may be based on past experiences or situations.) If older, how old? (Actually put a chronological age on the thought.)
- How do you feel about where your thoughts lead you?
- Do you gravitate toward certain feelings based on your thoughts?
- Are you judging the thoughts and yourself in the process?
- Do the thoughts tend to be true or valid?
- Do you recognize that there are other ways/alternative explanations of interpreting your thoughts and consider all aspects of a challenging situation in a balanced way?
- How could you problem solve so that you make choices that feel meaningful and are in line with your values and goals?
- How do you want to behave, and what kinds of actions will make that possible?

Once you and your child have had a chance to practice stepping back and looking more objectively at the way you think, you can begin to evaluate your thoughts and feelings about eating and exercise and try to understand them better together. Later on, we'll learn to identify, reframe, lean into, and defuse all kinds of thoughts that are preventing your child from achieving her goals.

Power cards can make this process concrete, and together we'll design one in Chapter 4. First, however, you and your child must become more aware of thoughts and feelings and more mindful of decision making by going through the aforementioned series of questions. You will both readily recognize that *thoughts are not facts.* Although at times, they can be very convincing.

STRATEGY 4

BE PRESENT

Purposefully Accept Whatever Shows Up

We explored how the mind has "a mind of its own" and how we can't control incoming thoughts, as hard as we may try. Learning to be present through mindfulness activities helps to tame the mind so there's space between the thinking and doing. Pema Chödrön, a Buddhist nun who wrote numerous books on mindfulness, describes it as creating space between the "craving" and "grabbing." Mindfulness alters our habitual responses by having us take a pause, so we can think about the decisions we want to make about our eating and exercise behaviors. When we purposefully take a moment to tune in to our hunger, we get the chance to actually taste our food rather than devouring it as we may have formerly done.

There tends to be confusion about what mindfulness is and why it's helpful. One popular definition of mindfulness, expressed by Jon Kabat-Zinn, is "paying attention in a particular way: on purpose, in the present moment, and nonjudgmentally."[7] In a nutshell, mindfulness is simply *fully* paying attention to what you are doing without judgment. It's described as a state and not a trait.[8] People are not inherently mindful; they must practice mindfulness.

Because life is so busy and you and your child are inundated with many tasks and responsibilities on a daily basis, you both may naturally go on autopilot. Think about how many times you enter a room to do something and notice that you forget what it is that you set out to accomplish. Or you sit down for a meal, and, before you know it, your plate is clean and you can't even remember eating the food. Or you are about to leave the shower, and you cannot recall if you washed your face or not. This is because you are not *fully* paying attention. This happens to your child, as

18

well! Unless you and your child, make a concerted effort to give your attention *fully*, you may miss out on some critical thoughts and feelings that affect your health behaviors, both positively and negatively.

People can practice a variety of mindfulness-based activities, such as yoga, tai chi, guided imagery, mindfulness-based stress reduction, mindfulness-based cognitive therapy, and meditation. Many evidence-based research studies have shown that mindfulness practices are helpful. Mindfulness is known to change the structure of the brain, facilitate a higher capacity for working memory, decrease mind wandering, and improve focus. It improves blood pressure, immune response, and sleep and is an effective strategy for managing chronic pain, fibromyalgia, rheumatoid arthritis, eating disorders, and weight issues. It helps with regulation of emotions and emotional processing, decreases levels of the stress hormone cortisol, decreases depression, and assists with body awareness, self-awareness, and acquiring compassion.[9]

In 2012, 477 scientific journal articles verified the effectiveness of mindfulness and meditative practices.[10] They have proven effective for kids and teens and assist with focusing and attention, executive functioning, sleep, emotional regulation, stress reduction, aggressive behavior, anxiety, and social skills/behaviors.[11] A recent study shows that mindfulness also helps prevent obesity in children by stopping impulses to overeat.[12]

Particularly for kids and teens who are digitally connected for much of their days, mindfulness is essential. The average teen sends and receives more than three thousand text messages a month.[13] Time to "just be," without constant stimulation and distractions, is hard to come by. Mindfulness has been compared to strength training for the mind. By engaging in the practice, your child's brain becomes bigger, stronger, and better equipped to handle challenges.

You can adapt mindfulness exercises to fit kids and teens at different ages and abilities. You could introduce mindfulness through your child's environment (awareness of objects and daily activities), their body (awareness of the senses, movement, or breath), meditation (awareness of their thinking process), and visualization (such as envisioning a bucket or jar of emotions, a bubble filled with thoughts and feelings, or checking in on a personal "weather report").[14] User-friendly guided meditations are earmarked at the end of each chapter. In general, activities should be clear, manageable, and engaging, taking into consideration where kids and teens are developmentally. There are also some good mindfulness apps for kids and teens, such as Insight Timer; Stop, Breathe and Think; Smiling Mind;

19

and Take a Break! (see Resources for a full list).

Your child may report feeling relaxed after a mindfulness exercise. Although not the goal of mindfulness, calmness can be a welcome by-product.[15] All thoughts and feelings are welcome; we don't aim them in any particular direction. Just *be* with whatever presents itself. The objective is to "just be" with it all—the comfortable, the uncomfortable, and the neutral.

A systematic, daily practice of mindfulness will help train your and your child's brains to "focus your attention on what's actually going on around you and inside of you."[16] It will help your child gain concentration as well as awareness of the full array of thoughts, feelings, and sensations that show up for him. This will allow him to create space so he can make more mindful, value-based decisions. He will learn to step back and avoid making assumptions about the way he thinks and feels and pay keen attention to all that is being presented to him. These concepts will first be described in general and then applied specifically to his eating and exercise behaviors.

EXERCISE: Practicing Mindfulness

Have your child practice these three behaviors, first mindlessly and then mindfully, and record the differences. The tasks can be accomplished on different days if need be.

1. **MINDLESSLY:** Go outside and take a quick walk down the block and back.
   MINDFULLY: Take a slow, leisurely walk down the block, being aware of your senses and surroundings. Pay attention to what you are seeing, hearing, smelling, etc.

2. **MINDLESSLY:** Take a quick shower.
   MINDFULLY: Take a slower shower, paying attention to the full experience, including all the tasks being accomplished and the accompanying physical sensations. Notice as you wash your hair and skin the experience of the water cascading down your body, your body temperature, etc.

3. **MINDLESSLY:** Walk into a room in your house, take a quick glance, and then exit that room.
   MINDFULLY: Walk into the same room and take the time to notice the room fully. Glance at the furniture, all the items throughout the room, all the shapes, sizes, and colors.

Then, ask him to jot down some notes on when he mindfully engaged in the activity.

- How did it feel to take this approach?
- Did you notice anything different from the experience of accomplishing it mindlessly as opposed to mindfully?
- What specifically did you notice that you didn't necessarily pay attention to before? What were you possibly missing out on by approaching it mindlessly?
- How do you think this could apply to your eating and exercise behaviors (for example, overeating because of eating quickly and mindlessly, or being mindful of how your body feels when you're exercising so you don't injure yourself)?

When your child is fully engaged in mindful eating and exercise behaviors, he will be able to notice such things as his cues around food, satiety, his triggers and urges to eat certain foods, how movement makes his body feel, and other key components that are essential for healthful behavior over the long term. Eating mindfully can also facilitate greater satisfaction from eating, because he is tuning in to every taste and moment of pleasure associated with the food and eating.

By recognizing and accepting the array of thoughts, feelings, and physical sensations that come up around eating, he can cope with them in a caring and compassionate way. Cultivating empathy and loving kindness can help disrupt cycles of overeating and the inevitable guilt and shame that result. As opposed to struggling with his thoughts, feelings, and sensations, he will learn to accept them.

STRATEGY 5

BE COMFORTABLE WITH BEING UNCOMFORTABLE

Challenge Your Urges

Ever since she was born, your child may have been taught that she should be in a "happy" state of mind. If she finds herself "unhappy," she may think that it is "bad" for her, there is something "wrong" with her, and she ought to transform her thoughts and feelings to ensure that she is "happy" and "okay." The underlining sentiment is that the "happier," more comfortable thoughts and feelings are preferred and the only ones that are truly acceptable. These are sentiments she has heard repeatedly throughout her life. She probably heard it from you, others she interacts with, and the media at large. You are not to blame for repeating the message; that's all you heard, too.

Search the Internet and you'll find numerous articles and blogs that tell you five, ten, twelve, twenty, and many more ways to gain happiness, implying that there are universal ways to define and achieve happiness. Does that make sense, considering we are all distinct, unique human beings with varied makeups, needs, and desires? Also, does that mean that the other side of happiness is depression? Then surely being unhappy is undesirable and threatening, right? Not so.

We are caught in "the happiness trap" (this is also the title of an enlightening book written by Russ Harris that focuses on ACT skills). What often seems as if it will make us happy ultimately makes us unhappy, because we get caught up in the struggle with our thoughts and the chase to find happiness. "Don't worry, be happy" is a nice mantra, but it is unrealistic and unattainable to expect to be happy all the time. For one, what is "happy"? It is not clear how this is defined and how it gets evaluated. For another, what exactly are we striving for? To never have unhappy or uncomfortable thoughts and/or feelings? The reality is that we cannot just deny, avoid, or get rid of our thoughts and feelings even though we may desperately want to. They are part of who we fundamentally are and what make us human.

Do not take my word for it. Try it yourself. Think about something that you are currently concerned about that needs to get accomplished in the very immediate future. I want you to spend the rest of today and tomorrow trying to get rid of the concern. Good luck! You may have temporary moments of distraction or calm, but the worry is still present, because it is what is going on for you. It needs to be honored. Ignoring, rejecting, or neglecting parts of you, notably your thoughts and feelings, will not make you feel more empowered and confident but undoubtedly more ashamed, sad, and disappointed. The other issue to consider is when less-favorable thoughts and feelings get cut off, the more-favorable ones get cut off, as well.

Uncomfortable thoughts and feelings are natural. If we deny that array of emotions, we are not honoring ourselves fully. I share the sentiment with my clients that we are not kids at a candy store, afforded with the choice of just selecting the candy we like and leaving the less desirable candy behind. We cannot simply select the thoughts and feelings we "prefer" to have because they feel better. *All* thoughts and feelings have value, are worth noting, contribute to who we are, and provide us with insight into the way we function and behave.

22

Still, we demonize certain thoughts, avoid them, and want to rid ourselves of them because that is what we are taught to do and what makes the most sense based on our human instincts. If we feel something is physically uncomfortable, we adjust to find comfort. Why shouldn't we apply the same strategy to our thoughts and feelings? Unfortunately, the strategy just doesn't work the same way. In trying over and over again to get rid of them, we're left with frustration when they still exist.

The only things we can truly control are our actions. But it will be difficult to change behaviors if you accept negative thoughts and self-criticism as facts. *We are bigger than our thoughts, and they do not get to define who we are. We get to define who we are, and we want our behavior to be based on our integrity and fundamental values.*

The mind naturally gravitates to the past, which often evokes regret and guilt (in the extreme resulting in depression), and the future, which often evokes worry and fear (in the extreme resulting in anxiety). The hardest state to secure is the present moment. When we get caught in the past or future, we lose sight of all the beauty the present has to offer. The challenge is to stay here, right now, mindfully.

EXERCISE: Being with Whatever Shows Up

Select a snack or food that your child tends to crave or overeat—for example, let's say potato chips. (For this exercise, try to select a food that does not melt when you place it in your mouth.) Complete each of the following steps for one to two minutes (you can carry this out with your child in order to share the experience):

- Open a small bag of potato chips.
- Take a large handful of chips and put them in a bowl.
- Hold the bowl of chips. Look at the chips and notice their elements: all the curves, colors, and shapes.
- Smell the chips. Fully take in their aroma.
- Touch the chips and notice their varied textures. Outline the shapes with your fingers.
- Put *one* chip in your mouth but do not chew or swallow it. Take time to fully taste the chip and experience all its flavors. Note whether it is salty, sweet, sour, or bitter. Do the same with four more chips, one at a time.
- Take the rest of the chips and throw them into the garbage.

This exercise will challenge your child to eat mindfully (slowly, intentionally, and paying attention) and sit with the probable craving of more chips. Let her sit with whatever shows up and explore the following:

1. What was it like to eat the chips mindfully?

    _____

    _____

    _____

    _____

2. Did you notice anything about the chips or your response to them that you hadn't noticed before?

    _____

    _____

    _____

    _____

3. What did you notice in regard to your general mood, bodily sensations, thoughts, and feelings?

    _____

    _____

    _____

    _____

4. What thoughts, feelings, and sensations are you experiencing with your craving for more chips?

    _____

    _____

    _____

    _____

5. Are you having a thought or feeling about throwing out the chips? Is it lingering? Changing over time?

    _____

    _____

    _____

    _____

Enforce that your child's discomfort is understandable because she is challenging herself and going out of her comfort zone. Acknowledge that the craving may be eliciting uncomfortable thoughts, feelings, and sensations now but that it will pass if she stays with all that comes up, rides it out, and acclimates herself to the discomfort. Reinforce that you are present to support her through it.

Space needs to be created so that we can thoughtfully process the situation and make mindful decisions on behalf of our health. There's a need for increased awareness, since, as a study has verified, we make about two hundred food-related decisions each day.[17]

CREATE SPACE

Process Thoughts and Actions with Purpose

Most individuals I work with report that when they overeat, they go from "zero to ten" automatically and don't usually remember having any thoughts in between experiencing the urge ("I want this food") and the doing (eating the food). They express that it just happens. During and after the incident, they are typically left feeling angry and frustrated. They experience shame and self-loathing because, from their perspective, they couldn't be more mindful and control their behavior. We have all been there. Space needs to be created so that we can thoughtfully process the situation and make mindful decisions on behalf of our health.

Creating space between the urge and the doing requires that we pace ourselves, observe ourselves, and be curious about ourselves. *All thoughts and feelings that show up in the process are okay; it is how we act on them that is our choice.*

According to ACT, we need a multielement approach to improve our circumstances. First, we need to pay attention to the present. This can be successfully practiced through mindfulness. As noted, mindfulness requires putting concerted effort into paying attention to what is happening now and being present with your eating and exercise behaviors as well as your thoughts and feelings toward food.

After mindfulness, another element of creating space is acceptance. Acceptance is your child's willingness to accept his uncomfortable thoughts and feelings about his health and weight challenges. The consideration isn't the degree to which he likes or doesn't like the thoughts and feelings but rather his willingness to be with whatever shows up. Part of acceptance is also his willingness to take a look at himself and evaluate who he is and how he functions. Throughout this book there will be steps for him to further learn about his thoughts, feelings, and behaviors in regard to his health. Value identification, another principle (covered in Chapter 2), will compel him to pursue his health and weight goals and objectives.

Defusion is another ACT principle that speaks to letting thoughts be what they are—just thoughts and not necessarily facts. If our minds tell us we'll fail, we should give up, and that maintaining a healthful practice is too hard to sustain, we can recognize that these are merely thoughts, and we don't have to "fuse" with them so that they do become fact. (See the next exercise, Mind over Muffin). Committed action, another ACT principle, speaks to committing and taking direct action toward your eating and exercise behaviors and goals. Many individuals get caught up in "trying" to take action. The actual doing is what facilitates change, not the trying to do.

———

EXERCISE: Mind over Muffin

Help your child distance himself from (defuse and reframe) self-sabotaging thoughts (you can role-play with him):

> **INSTEAD OF SAYING:** "I will only have one bite of the muffin."
> **REFRAME TO SAY:** "I am having the thought that I will have only one bite of the muffin."

> **INSTEAD OF SAYING:** "I need to have the muffin now!"
> **REFRAME TO SAY:** "I am having the thought that I need to have the muffin now."

> **INSTEAD OF SAYING:** "I should eat the muffin because everyone else is eating one."
> **REFRAME TO SAY:** "I am having the thought that I should eat the muffin because everyone else is eating one."

This mindfulness exercise illustrates how your child can create space in his thinking, defuse and/or reframe it, so that he can effectively process his thoughts and choose how he wants to behave in response to them. Remembering "mind over muffin" may result in his having half a muffin, a mini muffin, or no muffin at all. As long as he is eating mindfully and thoughtfully, he is practicing healthful eating behavior.

26

BAD FOOD, BAD PERSON

Understand the Way Language and Frame of Reference Impact Thoughts

ACT is grounded in Relational Frame Theory (RFT), which highlights the power of language in categorizing the things around us and, therefore, determining how we approach the world.[18] For example, if I held up an index card with the word *candy* written on it, you would most likely have a frame of reference in mind. If your favorite candy is taffy, you might imagine a gooey, sticky, cherry-flavored taffy bar. Another person might think of a chocolate bar loaded with caramel and peanuts.

Based on your personal frame of reference, you would visualize your candy, envision how it tastes, and maybe even have a saliva response driving your desire to have your candy in the here and now. You might also compare your candy with others' favorites and hold the impression that your candy is better than theirs and that some people clearly have no taste in candy.

Another way to illustrate frame of reference is to look at how we attach meaning to words. If you repeat a word over and over rapidly, it loses some or most of its meaning. Say the word *witch*. When you first bring it up, you think of a haggard, horrid, scary woman flying on a broomstick like you remember from *The Wizard of Oz*. Repeat *witch* rapidly again and again, "witch," "witch," "witch." Repeat it fifty times over (try it!)—you'll notice it loses most of its meaning and becomes just a sound. Our emotional response to the word *witch* comes from the associations surrounding the definition we learned.[19]

Because of our frames of reference, we evaluate and define the foods we eat and our eating and exercise behaviors. We are exposed to thinking about certain foods as "junk" food, "bad" food, "clean" versus "dirty" foods, etc. The detriment of this language is that if a child is eating a "bad" food, it typically induces the thought and feeling that *she's* bad because she is eating bad food. This thinking perpetuates a cycle of guilt and shame and demonizes foods that provide us with sustenance.

As a parent, you want to build up your child's self-acceptance, self-love, self-compassion, and integrity. To avoid the cycle of shame, self-loathing, and hopelessness, mindfulness around language also needs to be considered and practiced.

Being mindful of the way we use language to refer to, categorize, or frame food, eating, and exercise behaviors will help facilitate healthier thinking around food and exercise behaviors (see Chapter 3 for specific mindfulness-based eating skills).

 ## CHECK YOUR BAGGAGE

You have learned that our thoughts have a mind of their own and can at times be unwieldy, irrational, and a source of discomfort. Kids and teens may find it challenging to sit with their thoughts and feelings because of the extent of discomfort they evoke for them.

Likewise, it may be challenging for you to tolerate your child's discomfort. You may feel compelled to discontinue the exercises and thus reinforce the desire to avoid, distract, or get rid of uncomfortable thoughts. In fact, you may want to rid yourself of your negative thoughts, as well.

As uncomfortable as your child or you may be, it's critical to make the concerted effort to stay with whatever thoughts and feelings show up. Model these actions so that your child is encouraged to behave thoughtfully and mindfully, as well.

Mindfulness practices for kids and teens are not dramatically different than those for adults. Be sure to adapt exercises so that they are easy to understand, user-friendly, and engaging. Take note of your child's body language and expressive language to gauge whether your child is engaged.

Be open to making adjustments as you see fit to include creativity, imagination, and humor or whatever else speaks to your child. Be sure to practice flexibility in your approaches and behaviors that you want your child to emulate.

 ## REVIEW

Our minds buzz, loop, and play games, and often we are left with having thoughts about our thoughts and feelings about our feelings. Understanding how the mind functions and starting a mindful practice will help your child make more thoughtful decisions regarding eating and exercise behaviors.

To facilitate mindful, healthful behaviors, be aware that the mind:

- Actively and constantly processes information
- Rationalizes
- Can buzz, loop, and play games
- Tries to control thoughts in order to protect us
- Layers on more thoughts and feelings
- Can be slowed down
- Has the ability to create space between feeling and acting
- Can learn to be more comfortable with being uncomfortable
- Has the ability to purposefully and intently take notice
- Can learn to defuse from thoughts
- Has the ability to engage in self-refection and engage as an observer
- Evaluates foods based on our language and frames of reference.

 MINDFULNESS EXERCISE: Being Open to Mind and Body

See page 218 for the mindfulness exercise that corresponds to this chapter, and refer to page 217 for instructions on accessing the audio.

Connecting with Values

My fifteen-year-old daughter, Maya, struggles with her weight and fitting in because she looks and feels different than the other girls. For her cousin's wedding last year, she lost 10 pounds. She put effort into eating healthily and exercising. I was so proud, and she felt so good about her accomplishment. Fast-forward four months later, and we're right back where we started. I don't know how to get her back on track.

—KAREN, PARENT

My son gets annoyed with me when I bring up his weight. He says he doesn't care. I can't imagine, being as overweight as he is, that he really doesn't care; that's just impossible. It worries me that he actually may not care. If he did, he probably would do something about it.

—BRETT, PARENT

THIS CHAPTER IS ALL ABOUT rethinking exercise and eating in terms of kids and teens' values—what is really important to them in the short and long term. Simultaneously, the strategies in this chapter will guide kids and teens to define what health means to them. I must stress, what is important to adults is often totally irrelevant to kids and teens. On many fronts, the world of kids and teens can be inscrutable to adults. Here you are given the opportunity to understand that your child may have motives for getting and staying healthy separate from yours. You can become aware of what drives your child, and you can make efforts to tap into those motivations and honor your child's reasons.

What does it mean to have values? This is a poorly understood concept. Often we can feel that our values have been forced on us, because they are so often programmed and preached. As children, we discover the magic of play, the delights of the senses, and the warm glow of love, but we are rarely afforded the same organic opportunity to unearth the sacred vitality of our personal values. Values are derived from the ability to assign personal importance to certain aspects of our life—the art of valuation. The word itself implies worth, the ability to assess the meaning of our choices and desires. By teaching your child to identify core values, prioritize them, problem solve through them, and formulate healthful choices, you are teaching your child to invest in a life that has deep meaning.

It is important to identify our core values, because these are what we treasure in life, what make our lives meaningful. Examples of core values include family, friendship, compassion, and integrity. You can help your children assess the values they have been taught and evaluate whether they are values that they personally hold dear. Discuss whether the acquired values (from you, society, etc.) are ones to which they aspire. Decisions often come up in life, particularly relative to health, that may create conflict due to two or more important values operating at the same time. For example, your children must make decisions about whether they will exercise that day (value of health) or whether they will study because they have a big test coming up (value of education/knowledge); whether they will eat the second chocolate chip cookie (value of health) or say no to the aunt who made them (family values). They will soon discover that they can effectively problem solve through these decisions.

I will give you the inside scoop on the most common reasons kids and teens identify for wanting to exercise and eat healthily, based on my research. You'll discover what motivates them to make healthy changes and maintain them—these factors being their relationships, general health, fitness level, physical comfort, level of self-acceptance and self-love, and their freedom and independence. Because unhealthful eating, lack of exercise, and other counterproductive behaviors may have become part of a daily routine, this chapter focuses on the concept of "practice," a key component of healthy living and a theme that is at the heart of this book.

This chapter also outlines barriers to healthful eating and exercising. Just because kids and teens may feel stuck does not mean that they will always feel that way; it is within their power to develop new practices that will help them become who they want to be over time. Kids can learn to make decisions on a daily basis that demonstrate a commitment to who they want to be and the values they feel are at their core.

As with adults, kids and teens need to remind themselves regularly *why* they have made the decision to invest in their health. Identifying core values relating to health will help them continually remember why they want to continue their practice. Some of the core values that will be described more fully in this chapter include relationships, physical health, physical fitness, physical comfort, self-acceptance/self-love, and freedom/independence. Formulating values and specific eating and exercising goals will enable your child to remain focused for the long run. At times this task may be challenging, and just like anything that it is important, it will require diligence, practice, and purposeful effort.

To identify key values relevant to kids and teens, there are several exercises that you can do with your child. These speak to the personal cost that less-than-optimal health may have for your child: relationship costs, health costs, fitness costs, physical comfort costs, self-acceptance/self-love costs, and loss of freedom/independence. The exercises also include self-assessments to encourage kids and teens to think about how and why they take care of themselves and how satisfied they are with their health. Together, you can learn why good health is important to your child.

Integrating a new practice driven by core values is a powerful cognitive shift and one that will be reinforced throughout this book. One of the central tenets of this practice is learning to continually find new and compelling reasons for reaching for something, especially when the goal is a lifetime project that has no beginning, middle, or end. You will guide your child to think of motivation and commitment in a new way.

STRATEGY 8

WHY BOTHER?

Understand Why Connecting to Your Values Is Important

You are probably wondering how willing your child is to invest in healthy living. You may question how much he wants this for himself or cannot understand why he is not compelled to make changes in the ways you think he ought to. You may be the type of person who has a hard time relating to this reluctance—perhaps when you have a goal in mind, you instantly go for it without hesitation. Alternatively, maybe you can relate to procrastination, reluctance, hooking onto self-defeating thoughts and feelings, and struggling to find a sense of purpose yourself.

If you reach the conclusion that your child is not readily making healthful changes, you may think that it's because he doesn't care. But it's likely that he is secretly in angst over his health behaviors and actually cares much more than he shows. He is struggling to find the "right" way, because he may have already tried various approaches and has yet to feel successful, or he wants to commit to the value of health but may not yet feel deeply connected to it.

Any behavior can become a self-fulfilling prophecy. If your child thinks he is viewed negatively, he may feel frustrated and inclined to act out behaviors that are in line with that perception of him. He remains hopeless and stuck—he cannot find his way out of that thinking and functioning, thus perpetuating the cycle and keeping him in the same position over time. Helping your child understand his core values is a good way to get him to tap into his willingness, motivation, what is meaningful to him, and what he stands for.

Here are some facts about values to convey to your child:

1. **VALUES REFLECT HOW YOUR CHILD IDEALLY WANTS TO LIVE AND WHAT DIRECTION HE WILL TAKE IN ORDER TO DO SO.** There is no beginning, middle, or end to discovering his values; the process is ongoing. For example, if he values education and learning, he will never stop learning. He will never reach the point of "I have learned enough." Every moment can be a moment of opportunity for him, whether he is perusing social media, studying directly from a textbook, or going to a museum to see an exhibit. Health works in the same way. He will have opportunities throughout his day to acknowledge his values, whether choosing to brush his teeth, deciding to walk the stairs instead of taking the elevator, or electing to eat the protein-enriched multigrain waffles rather than the regular processed ones.

2. **VALUES ARE "ABOUT WHAT YOU WANT TO DO, NOT ABOUT HOW YOU WANT TO FEEL.**[20] "I want to feel confident" is not a value. To get to the value, have your child ask himself: If I felt confident, then what would I be doing differently? The "value" here might be connecting with friends or being more invested in his education.

3. **VALUES AND GOALS ARE DIFFERENT.** Values are actions ("participate in physical activity") or qualities of action that can be stated as adverbs ("eat healthily").[21] Values are what drive your child's goals and the actions that he will inevitably take. Goals tend to be specific, distinct steps that he can attain.[22] He *can* go through the process of checking off goals when they are complete. For

example, "I will limit snacking to one time per day" or, "I will jog three miles three times per week." He *cannot* check off values—they are ongoing and enduring. Goals are steps that he would take along the way of moving toward his values. For example, if one of his values is learning, a goal might be to do well on his biology test. He can take steps to achieve that by, say, making an outline of all his notes three days prior to the exam, reviewing with friends two days before the exam, and having you quiz him the day before the test. The value of learning will extend beyond the biology test and will lead him to follow a similar process (or one that may work even better for him) on his trigonometry exam. If he doesn't highly value learning, maybe he'll check off that he received a decent grade in biology but not put as much time and effort into his trigonometry exam.

4. **VALUES ARE PERSONAL.** To gauge whether a value is truly important to your child, you may ask him, "If no one knew you were doing this, would it still be important to you?" So, for example, if *you* value compassion, you would probably say that even if no one knew you were being compassionate toward your child, it would still be important to you.[23]

5. **IN YOUR PAIN YOU FIND VALUES, AND IN YOUR VALUES YOU FIND YOUR PAIN.**[24] Because values are considered deeply personal choices that hold great meaning, your child may experience pain associated with his values. For example, if he values personal connection but gets into an argument with his friend at school, and they begin ignoring one another, he will undoubtedly feel disappointed and sad about the current state of their relationship.

6. **YOUR CHILD MAY ACQUIRE VALUES FOR MANY DIFFERENT REASONS.** He may have adopted them from you or your family; they may be influenced by what he thinks is expected of him; they can be instilled by culture or society or because of who he fundamentally is and what his desires are. Whatever the reason, his values will reflect what is important to your child.

7. **A FAILURE TO FOCUS ON VALUES DOESN'T CANCEL OUT HIS VALUES.** Even if he didn't have many moments of learning over the course of the day because he was occupied with video games, that doesn't mean that he doesn't value learning. He is just choosing not to

exercise that value in the moment. Nothing can take away his core values. They are present even if they are not being directly acted upon.

8. **THERE ARE BARRIERS TO VALUE-CONSISTENT BEHAVIOR.** These can be broken up into general categories, including but not limited to: societal barriers (e.g., thinness being idealized in magazines and on TV), thoughts and feelings (e.g., black-and-white thinking that circumstances can never change), behavioral barriers (e.g., a control strategy such as severly restricting eating as opposed to working through cravings and urges), and being unclear about what one's values actually are (e.g., losing weight is a goal with an end point and an inevitable contemplation of *Now what?* once the weight is lost, but goals are more likely to be productive and achievable when they are guided by values.[25] If weight loss is not guided by valuing health, it is less likely to be achieved or sustained over time).[26]

Valuing health encompasses a lot more than just eating well and exercising. It also includes daily self-care (brushing teeth, showering, going for annual doctor's visits, etc.). Consider all these factors when your child evaluates how meaningful this value is.

EXERCISE: Getting in Touch with the Value of Health

Ask your child to do the following: Have him close his eyes and take five minutes to think about how much time he spends in the course of a day taking care of his health.

Health is multifaceted and includes eating healthfully, engaging in physical activity, and maintaining personal hygiene, sleep hygiene, emotional and psychological health, and social health. You and your child can list all the ways in which you take care of your physical and emotional well-being.

It will become clear from doing this exercise that valuing health is all-encompassing: It consists of many elements and acts that are truly important to you.

AT ALL COSTS

Assess the Cost of Unhealthful Behaviors

Your child experiences consequences when her health is not being adequately addressed. In order for her to make her health a priority and implement goals accordingly, she needs to get a sense of how her good health, or lack of it, personally affects her and what changes she would like to see happen. For example, she may ask herself, "Do I have the energy to run around the basketball court the way that I want to? Am I physically healthy according to my doctor's report during my annual exam? Do I feel good about myself?" Taking personal responsibility for her health is critical.

EXERCISE: The Costs of Being Overweight

In this exercise, your child will think about what the costs of being overweight have been for her. Awareness is often the impetus for change. If she recognizes that she is not living the life she wants to lead, it can prompt her to want to make changes, particularly when she has the resources in place to go about doing so. She can complete this exercise with you or independently.

1. **RELATIONSHIP COSTS:** Summarize the effects of being overweight on your relationships. Do you tend to avoid socializing because of thoughts that you will be rejected, excluded, or made fun of? Do you not want to eat around others? Or do you avoid activities with friends when there is food or physical activity involved?

   _____

   _____

   _____

2. **HEALTH COSTS:** Summarize the effects on your health. Do you get ill more often? Is your weight impacting your sleep? Do you feel tired most of the time? According to your doctor, has it impacted your blood pressure or cholesterol level? Do you have any other health issues?

   _____

   _____

   _____

3. **FITNESS COSTS**: Summarize the effects on your physical fitness. Do you have a difficult time playing sports because of moving at a slower pace than you would like to? Do you have difficulty being active in general? Do you have difficulty catching your breath when you exert yourself?

_____

_____

_____

_____

4. **PHYSICAL COMFORT COSTS**: Summarize the effects on your physical comfort. Do you generally feel uncomfortable in your clothing? Are you uncomfortable fitting into certain seats? Are you uncomfortable when you're doing certain physical activities?

_____

_____

_____

_____

5. **SELF-ACCEPTANCE/SELF-LOVE COSTS**: Summarize the effects on your self-acceptance/self-love. Have you put time and energy into diets, exercise regimens, and quick fixes but had difficulty maintaining changes in the long run? Are you spending an extensive amount of time thinking about food, diet, and exercise? Do you feel frustrated and hopeless about your situation? Do you frequently experience shame, guilt, and self-deprecating thoughts in regard to your health and weight challenges? Do you blame yourself for not getting it "right" and not having the ability to make long-term change?

_____

_____

_____

_____

6. **COSTS OF FREEDOM/INDEPENDENCE**: Summarize the effects on your freedom/independence. Are you inhibited from buying new clothes? Do you compromise on the styles or type of clothing you buy? Are you missing out on events you want to go to or activities you want to try? Do you avoid participating in sports teams or other types of recreational activities such as swimming because of having to wear a bathing suit or gym clothing? Does it keep you

from doing the things that you want to and from being part of the larger community at school or in other settings?

_____

_____

_____

_____

7. Which cost has had the biggest impact on your life? How do you feel about acknowledging that this is the case? Are you willing to put in the time and effort on an ongoing basis if it results in living the life you truly want to lead?

_____

_____

_____

_____

Your child may not realize the significant costs of her behaviors and how they may influence various parts of her life that are important to her. As you read this book, you will be able to teach her skills to carry out the changes she needs to make.

STRATEGY 10

SEE VALUES IN ACTION

Pinpoint Why Healthful Living Is Important to You

Values should influence how your child chooses to behave. Behavior should not be controlled by others or based on things he might be receiving from others—for example, valuing good health because it will allow him to be "noticed" and "complimented." These outcomes are possible but cannot be guaranteed.

Values have no contingencies. They are about taking action and striving to reach goals that direct you toward your core value. For example, take your value of showing compassion for your child. If you were to fully engage in that value, you would aim to be compassionate no matter what; even if you were seething because your child disrespected you and gave you attitude, you would be compassionate and helpful if, say, he fell and hurt himself. Even though you may not feel especially connected to the value at the moment, you would show him compassion and not wait until he is respectful and likable again.

Your child may have formed his overeating habits for a variety of reasons (e.g., his physiological, emotional, or social makeup, what he learned, etc.). In order to change these habits, he needs to feel that change is warranted, that there are compelling reasons to do so, and that he has the resources available to him to be able to carry out the change.

———

EXERCISE: Why Is Healthful Living Important to Me?

Have your child fill out this worksheet to tap into what he fundamentally desires that connects him to healthful living. He should check off the statements that apply to him and fill in additional desires. *Remind him that health underpins all the values he holds.* For example, if he is not feeling well, then he cannot participate in his playoff game (fitness, freedom/independence), go to the movies with his friends (relationships), or celebrate his great-grandmother's ninetieth birthday (relationships).

RELATIONSHIPS:

- ❏ I want to improve my connection with my friends (e.g., have been avoiding them because of shame).
- ❏ I want to improve my connection with family (e.g., arguments around eating behavior).
- ❏ I want to go with friends to activities where food is present.
- ❏ I want to eat with others.
- ❏ I want to attend social events where physical activities are involved.
- ❏ I want to engage in physical activities with friends.
- ❏ I want to _____.

HEALTH:

- ❏ I want to get sick less often.
- ❏ I want to sleep better.
- ❏ I want to be less tired.
- ❏ I want to get a clean bill of health from my doctor.
- ❏ I want to _____.

FITNESS:

- ❏ I want to be stronger.
- ❏ I want to be more energetic.
- ❏ I want to be more agile and flexible when I _____.

❏ I want to be able to move at a faster pace when I am

_____.

❏ I want to _____.

PHYSICAL COMFORT:

❏ I want to fit more comfortably in my clothing.
❏ I want to be able to go anywhere and not be restricted because of the space I need to accommodate my size.
❏ I want to feel more comfortable when I'm engaging in

_____.

❏ I want to _____.

SELF-ACCEPTANCE/SELF-LOVE:

❏ I want to stop wasting my time and money on quick fixes that leave me feeling _____.
❏ I want to have greater confidence in myself and my ability to

_____.

❏ I want to be less self-critical.
❏ I want to acknowledge and feel proud of myself for my accomplishments.
❏ I want to _____.

FREEDOM/INDEPENDENCE:

❏ I want to spend less time hyper-focusing on _____ (e.g., my next meal, when I will have time to exercise, etc.) and more time focusing on living my life meaningfully.
❏ I want to do more things than I used to do because _____ (e.g., eating large portions, overeating sweets, not exercising enough, etc.) is holding me back.
❏ I want to buy clothing that I like and that makes me feel proud.
❏ I want to be able to pick from a variety of different styles and types of clothing.
❏ I want to attend events of my choosing no matter what I'm required to wear.
❏ I want to try new activities.
❏ I want engage more in community and school activities.
❏ I want to _____.

Consider each of these. Which values do you hold? Check them off. Are there others that you would include? What are they? In order, which are most important and connect you with healthful living?

- ❏ Relationships
- ❏ Health
- ❏ Fitness
- ❏ Physical Comfort
- ❏ Self-Acceptance/Self-Love
- ❏ Freedom/Independence
- ❏ Other _____

This strategy will help your child identify why healthful eating and engaging in physical exercise are important to him. His values need to be what he selects as truly meaningful. As a parent, you may think that he should care about his health for the same reasons that you do. But each child is unique, and his individual reasons are valid, important, and the key to what will motivate him toward healthful living.

STRATEGY 11

WHOSE LIFE IS IT, ANYWAY?

Examine Which Values Are Yours

Your child has to contend with a lot when it comes to the way she looks, feels, and perceives herself. The pressure to conform and get validation from others will always be there. However, if your child has a good sense of her values and what is meaningful to her, she will be more likely to look within herself for validation.

Goals such as "I want to look good" are often propelled by the thinking "If I look good, others will like me" or "I want to be thinner and prettier to be accepted and sought after." These goals are problematic because they are contingent on others, subjective, not measurable, and often lead to shameful and self-defeating thoughts and feelings. It becomes a problem when "we *need* to look good on the outside in order to feel good about ourselves on the inside."[27]

When so much time is spent focusing on physical appearance and what others think, a negative impact on self-confidence is inevitable. It also takes valuable time away from other things, such as finding genuine ways to foster self-acceptance and self-love. With solid values in place, the focus goes from seeking the approval of others to something your child does for herself because she truly cares about herself.

She may not necessarily be in touch with what her values intrinsically are. She may be able to tell you generally what are important goals that she wants to achieve, but she may not readily identify the core values that propel those goals. Or she may complain that the adults in her life do not let her choose and that her values have to be in line with the values that her parents elect as important.[28] For example, you may have started an exercise regimen when you reached adulthood because of fearing osteoporosis, mortality, or any of number of things. Because of where your child is developmentally, she does not have the same fears that would compel her participation.

When I meet with parents, I always ask them how they approach healthy living with their families. Most often they tell me that they express to their children that they will live a long life, their organs will function better, and they will feel better about themselves. I respond by sharing where their children are developmentally and suggest that how they have been approaching the issue may not be tapping into the intrinsic values that will compel their children to make sustaining behavioral changes.

Kids and teens are generally far away from thinking about their mortality and typically feel invincible and indestructible. They are not thinking about their organs or "health" per se and tend to be consumed with thinking about their friends, school, and daily activities. Also, when talking about "feeling better about themselves," kids and teens most often do not want to address the way they feel or typically feel "fine" just the way they are. In reality, kids often get offended when and if parents suggest otherwise.

EXERCISE: Assess Your Healthy-Living Values

First, do this exercise on your own. Then do the same exercise with your child. Identify which of your personal values are linked to healthful living. Which of these were acquired? How have they been acquired (based on who you "should" or "must" be, influenced by family, culture, gender, society, etc.)? Which are personal to you? In what ways are they personal?

These values can overlap. For example, you might have been taught by your parents that physical activity is essential because most family vacations revolve around participating in some kind of physical activity. It is a value you acquired and one that is also personal?

RELATIONSHIPS: _____

PHYSICAL HEALTH: _____

PHYSICAL FITNESS: _____

PHYSICAL COMFORT: _____

SELF-ACCEPTANCE/SELF-LOVE: _____

FREEDOM/INDEPENDENCE: _____

OTHER: _____

Values that are personal to you may be very different from values personal to your child. Those will be the ones that inevitably stick with your child and will be self-sustaining, because your child will want to take personal responsibility for them. Her personal values will establish what she fundamentally cares about and represent what she wants to be about.

STRATEGY 12

GET UNSTUCK

Evaluate Your Current Behavior

By being overweight, your child is possibly perceived by others (and may perceive himself) as lazy, unmotivated, unwilling, or incapable of making healthful changes. If he is being labeled or labels himself, change may be harder to come by.

Being stuck gets in the way of your child following through and acting on behalf of his health values and goals. If there is "stuckness" between the knowing and the doing, there is a reason for it. In general, if kids and teens get labeled, they give up and are given up on. If your child is stuck, you can find out what is getting in his way and help facilitate effective change.

In order to get unstuck and start implementing healthful eating and fitness values and goals, kids and teens need to assess current behaviors. Have your child evaluate whether he is leaning *toward* his health values or *away* from them by the actions he is taking. Identify barriers to healthful living, effectively formulate goals, and problem solve when two competing values are presented.

EXERCISE: Assessing Current Health Behavior

Have your child complete the following exercise:

1. How satisfied are you with your health?

   _____

   _____

   _____

   _____

2. On a scale of 1 (not satisfied) to 5 (very satisfied), how satisfied are you with your:

   Physical Fitness: _____

   Eating Behaviors: _____

3. How are you acting on behalf of your health?

   Physical fitness: Are you exercising for at least sixty minutes a day, three times per week, including moderate or vigorous activity, muscle-strengthening activities such as gymnastics or push-ups, and bone-strengthening activities such as jumping rope or running (the recommended amount by the Centers for Disease Control and Prevention)? If not, how often are you exercising? What forms of exercise?

   _____

   _____

   _____

   _____

   Eating healthfully: Are you eating a well-balanced diet? Are you getting help with this? Do you snack more often than you would like to? Would you prefer to be eating other foods than the ones you are consuming? Are the portions that you are eating in line with healthful eating? (See the serving size chart on page 72.)

   _____

   _____

   _____

   _____

4. Barriers to healthful living:

My barriers to physical fitness are:

_____

_____

_____

_____

My barriers to eating healthfully are:

_____

_____

_____

_____

5. Goal setting (identify short-term, medium-range, and long-term goals):

In order to work toward physical fitness, I will commit to:

(Example: Participating in three fitness activities this week and establishing what activities I'm interested in and want to pursue on a weekly basis. I will try kickboxing, tennis, cycling, jogging, swimming, and Zumba.)

_____

_____

_____

_____

In order to work toward healthful eating, I will commit to:

(Example: Eating two snacks a day consisting of fruit and vegetables of my choice.)

_____

_____

_____

_____

These goals should be reevaluated at the end of each week to consider whether to continue or revise them.

EXERCISE: Competing Values

Often, two important values can be competing at the same time. In these situations, your child will most likely feel pulled in two directions and have uneasiness about making a decision. Something important to him will inevitably be compromised, which may leave him with some unsettling feelings.

An example of this is deciding to earmark Tuesday as an exercise day (health/physical-fitness value), but the debate-team meeting (education/ learning value) is scheduled for that same evening. Both are important, but neither can be rescheduled for that week, and your child doesn't want to give up either. Despite having to go back on the commitment for that specific health goal for that week, your child decides going to the debate-team meeting makes more sense because a local competition is coming up and he could use the practice.

At this point, black-and-white, all-or-nothing thinking may sneak in and dictate that he totally give up on the idea of working out that week. Instead, he could decide to engage in his value of participating in physical fitness in different ways. Perhaps it's proactively taking the stairs at school instead of riding the elevator, or opting to walk the dog all week.

In order to work through situations where competing values arise, ask your child to complete the following exercise:

1. Identify situations where you have competing values:

   _____
   _____
   _____
   _____

2. How you felt in that situation:

   _____
   _____
   _____
   _____

3. How you decided between the competing values and what you decided to do:

   _____
   _____
   _____
   _____

Going through this process allows your child to begin untangling "stuckness." The best way to do it is to continue acting on behalf of his values with consistency and concerted effort. Sometimes it will be easy, and other times will be more challenging. Remember, there is no list to check off, and there is no end point; health is an ongoing process that gets repeatedly worked on.

PRACTICE DOESN'T MAKE PERFECT, AND THAT'S OKAY

Commit to the Value of Health

When your child commits to healthy living, she engages in a continual practice of making choices and taking action on behalf of her values and what is important to her.[29] The goal of engaging in an ongoing practice is not to reach perfection or an ideal; it is to put your child on a path toward living a meaningful life.

There will be times of challenge, frustration, and slipups—it is bound to happen. These challenges are not necessarily a reflection of health not being important to your child, that she is not taking it seriously, or that she will inevitably give up on it all together. Rather, they reflect being human. We all slip up at times, even if unintentionally. We can always work to improve and enhance ourselves. The goal is not to change who we are fundamentally but to accept ourselves with our imperfections. It can be helpful to remind your child of three affirmations of well-being: "There's nothing wrong with you," "You have everything you need to succeed," and "You are whole and complete."[30]

EXERCISE: Committing to My Value of Health

The following is a letter your child can fill out to help ground her, get in touch with her values, and strengthen her commitment to the process.

My values are important to me because they help me to live a meaningful life, one that I am personally proud of. They lead me to act in ways that define what I stand for, who I am, and who I want to continue to be. I am committing to the value of health.

Every day as I go on my journey, I am going to have opportunities to exercise this value. I will seek out opportunities that will allow me to practice my commitment to health. Even if I have slipups along the way, it doesn't mean that my core value is canceled out. I will return to my value of health, set goals for myself, and act on behalf of my value whenever I can.

The value of health is important to me because:

_____
_____
_____
_____

Based on my value, I will carry out the following initial goals:
_____, _____, and
_____. Over time, I am committing to amending my goals and formulating new goals that are in line with my value.

As I go on my journey, there may be barriers along the way. Some barriers may include:

_____
_____
_____
_____

I'm going to address these barriers by using supports and resources:

_____
_____
_____
_____

When I reflect on my day, I see that I acted in the following ways, which are helping me express my value:

_____
_____
_____
_____

I choose health as a value and am proud of who I am and what I stand for. I am doing something meaningful for myself. This will be a continual journey with ups and downs specific to my experience. I will continue no matter what shows up, because it's important to me.

During and following slipups, offering support and extending empathy and compassion to your child encourage her to re-enroll in committed action toward her health values and goals. She will learn that through committed action, her circumstances can change and that she has the power to help facilitate that change.

 ## CHECK YOUR BAGGAGE

Your perception of your child's "willingness" to invest in healthful behaviors may provoke a whole host of feelings for you. Sometimes you have limited information and are left guessing based on your own set of perceptions and fears. Be mindful of these perceptions, and avoid acting out negatively. Recognize that although your child may outwardly appear to be lazy or unwilling, your child may need help connecting to the value of health in order to take committed action on it.

Guide kids and teens through the process of identifying what their personal reasons are for connecting to this value. They'll be more willing to work through this with you if they feel supported and you exhibit a caring nurturing, compassionate, and nonjudgmental posture. If they sense your disapproval of them or their choices, you run the risk of them distancing themselves from you.

You may have also formed opinions about what values they should hold regarding their health and what short-term, medium-range, and long-term goals they should put in place. You may also observe their own personal frustration and disappointment around this, which makes it even more painful for you, because you hate to see them in distress. You may be prompted to jump in and immediately state your opinions and structure your guidance around the way you think things should be done.

Instead, take the time to learn more about what drives them, what they want to be about, and what they want to stand for. Allow for their own set of values to drive their actions. If they feel they are being imposed upon, they are less likely to invest in and work toward their health and sustain the practice.

 ## REVIEW

This chapter provided you and your child with an overview of what values are and what purpose they serve. You explored the costs of being overweight and the impact it has. We discussed the values linked to healthful living and how to untangle "stuckness" by evaluating how satisfied you and your child are with behaviors exhibited.

Sustainable change is possible if you and your child set specific goals that are in line with the value of health.

Parents can:

- Convey the purpose of values. When values hold personal meaning to kids and teens, they positively drive behavior.
- Review the costs of being overweight.
- Identify why healthful living is personally important to kids and teens.
- Assess both current healthful behaviors as well as barriers to successfully carrying out kids and teens' values and goals.

 MINDFULNESS EXERCISE: Who You Want to Be

See page 219 for the mindfulness exercise that corresponds to this chapter, and refer to page 217 for instructions on accessing the audio.

3

Helping Kids and Teens Get to Know Themselves

I don't want to accept this about me. I want to be thin like my sister. Why did I have to get stuck with my mother's genes!?!

—RACHEL, AGE 14

I don't know what to do when my son Ellis heads over to the snack drawer after a huge lunch just a few hours before. I don't get how he could eat another thing after a meal like that. I'm stuffed. When a craving hits him, watch out, world, he's a man on a mission.

—SABRINA, PARENT

OUR MINDS CAN COMPEL US to believe that ignorance is bliss because of what we think we may discover about ourselves—something we fear may be too uncomfortable to bear. Rather than explore who we are, inclusive of our imperfections, we are driven to ignore ourselves. We avoid or defend against our traits that we disapprove of or would rather not have. But when trying to change behavior over the long term, knowledge and acceptance are vital.

Kids and teens can be their own private investigators into the way they think, feel, and behave. Using "the 4Ps" (predict, plan, put into action, and practice—explored in depth in Chapter 5) will allow them to know what to generally expect and will allow them to plan actions relative to their healthful goals. Cognitive-Behavioral Therapy (CBT), which was developed by Aaron T. Beck in the early 1960s, is the most research-based treatment for altering behavior to date. The CBT model proposes that our thinking impacts our feelings, which directly impact our behavior. It says that "when people learn to evaluate their thinking in a more realistic and adaptive way, they experience improvement in their emotional state and in their behavior."[31] In the early 2000s, Judith S. Beck expanded CBT to apply it to eating behavior.[32] Throughout this book, I use the CBT model to assist you in understanding how kids and teens' thoughts affect their feelings and, therefore, their eating and exercise behaviors. This treatment gives a road map on how to effectively help your child develop or improve healthful behaviors.

Everyone has cravings and self-sabotaging thoughts—they just vary from person to person. And even within your child, they shift regularly. Your child can get a good gauge of when these thoughts and cravings are influencing behaviors by getting to know them and being ready when anything comes up. Thoughts and feelings are what they are. Acceptance and nonjudgment makes us gentler and kinder to ourselves.

This chapter begins a process of self-evaluation to help kids and teens take personal responsibility for their own health. Using a number of self-assessment tools, kids and teens will identify their health history (e.g., reactions to cravings, willingness to change, etc.) and will learn more about their eating behaviors (i.e., cravings versus hunger, emotional eating, etc.).

The assessment process also covers other areas, including attitudes toward healthy eating and exercise, eating habits, hunger versus cravings, thirst, overeating, and other reasons kids and teens may engage in overeating. I provide guided exercises to enable them to document their feelings and their reactions to this process, to look at what they are eating and the thoughts, feelings, and behaviors associated with it, how hungry they feel they are throughout the day, and how this hunger may fluctuate.

After completing the assessments, you and your child will have a better sense of yourselves and the challenges you face.

STRATEGY 14

PERSONAL PI

Evaluate All That You Are

Have your child complete the following self-evaluation, in which he becomes his own private investigator. The aim is to raise his awareness regarding where he was in the past, where he is presently, and where he hopes to go based on committed action to this process.[33] It is a general gauge, and it is important to encourage him to answer candidly and to the best of his ability. The purpose of the evaluation is for him to gain self-awareness, which he will be able to achieve if he responds thoughtfully.

EXERCISE: Self-Evaluation

Ask your child to rate and evaluate his willingness to change, eating behaviors, hunger and cravings, and emotional eating.

WILLINGNESS LEVEL

In these scenarios, rate your willingness: 0 (not willing), 1 (slightly willing), 2 (moderately willing), or 3 (very willing).

How willing are you to adjust your eating and exercise habits? _____

How willing are you to prepare healthier choices or ask your parents or someone else for help with the preparation? _____

How willing are you to put in the time needed to exercise? _____

How willing are you to put in the effort to find a method of exercising or physical fitness that you will stick to? _____

How willing are you to tell relevant people that you are changing the way you eat? _____

How willing are you to experience uncomfortable thoughts and feelings in the course of improving your healthful eating and exercise behaviors? _____

EATING BEHAVIORS

Indicate how often you perform these: 0 (never), 1 (occasionally), 2 (moderately often), or 3 (very often).

How often do you eat standing up (or get out of your seat while you are eating)? _____

How often do you eat quickly and find yourself being one of the first ones at the table to finish their meal? _____

How often do you forget to notice every bite you are eating because you are distracted by other things (e.g., TV, electronics, etc.)? _____

How often are you frustrated or disappointed because you ate more than you intended to? _____

How often are you frustrated or disappointed because you intended to make healthier food choices? _____

How often do you feel it is unfair because it seems as if your friends or others are eating whatever or as much as they like? _____

How often do you feel deprived because you are not able to eat the things you like to eat? _____

How often do you think that committing to your health is just too hard? _____

How often do you feel that committing to healthful behavior is just not worth it? _____

HUNGER AND CRAVINGS

Indicate how often you experience these: 0 (never), 1 (occasionally), 2 (moderately often), or 3 (very often).

How often do you try to avoid your hunger or cravings and eat in anticipation of feeling hungry or that you'll have a craving? _____

How often do you think, I really need to eat something now?

_____

How often do you make excuses and rationalize why you're eating something or the amount you're choosing to eat? _____

How often are you unsure if you're really hungry or not? _____

How often are you confused whether you're hungry or thirsty?

_____

How often do you feel that only one type of food will satiate you and your hunger? _____

EMOTIONAL EATING

Indicate how often you experience these: 0 (never), 1 (occasionally), 2 (moderately often), or 3 (very often).

How often do you eat more than you ordinarily would when you're feeling . . .

Down, sad, or disappointed? _____

Nervous, worried, or anxious? _____

Lonely? _____

Angry, frustrated, or annoyed? _____

Bored? _____

Like procrastinating about doing something you know you should do? _____

Tired? _____

Physically unwell? _____

As part of an ongoing process, it is helpful for your child to keep a journal of his journey on a daily or weekly basis (or as often as he would like). Not all kids and teens like to write, and some find it a chore. If that's the case with your child, you can also suggest jotting down brief bullet points, using voice memos in his smartphone, or just talking it out with you or someone else he trusts. If he chooses to write, here is why it will be helpful for him and a general format that he may follow.

In the process of your child's journey toward healthful eating and exercise behaviors, a variety of thoughts and feelings will come up about the skills being learned, his relationship with others, and challenges that he is experiencing or that he anticipates. A journal is an effective way for him to express and process all of this. Journaling is helpful to:

- Explore the thoughts and feelings about what he is learning and experiencing on a regular basis.
- Express concerns, frustrations, and accomplishments.
- Evaluate his needs, goals, and progress.
- Get in touch with his feelings, which may not come naturally for him (it doesn't for most kids and teens).
- Feel supported through challenges.
- Reflect on his values, which will reinforce his willingness and motivation in the process.
- Openly express himself. It's private, confidential, and for his own personal use. It may prompt him to be more open to the process.
- Measure his progress over time.

Please encourage your child to write free-flowing thoughts. There is no need for him to pay attention to grammar, spelling, or punctuation. Keep in mind that this is a method to organize, process, and understand his thoughts and feelings more clearly. He should feel free to use the following prompts or the parts that he finds relate to him. He can write as much or as little as he likes. Some suggested topics include:

- What you are gaining awareness of or learning that you didn't know before?
- Of these, what stands out as being the most important to you?
- What specific values are operating for you as you go along in your journey?
- What specific goals are you working on? Have they changed? If yes, how?
- Have you noticed how you're feeling about yourself and what feelings are coming up? Has that shifted at all? How?
- Has anything shifted in your relationships with others? If yes, how and in what ways?
- What challenges are you confronted with? How do you feel you're handling them? What do you need to continue doing? Or do differently?
- Are you noticing your accomplishments? What are they?
- How are you feeling in general in regard to gaining awareness, learning, and committing to your health?

STRATEGY 15

THE CUPCAKE CONUNDRUM

Differentiate Among Hunger, Thirst, Desire, and Cravings

Many people have difficulty gauging when they're hungry and when they're not. There are differences between actual hunger and sensations that trick us into believing that they are hunger. When your child sits down for a meal, it is best for her not to come to the table ravenous. When she's that hungry, it is more likely that she'll overeat or binge, because her blood sugar may have plummeted. When she wants to eat, assess on a scale from 1 to 10 how hungry she actually is[34]:

1. Insatiably hungry
2. Seriously hungry
3. Stomach-growling hungry
4. Slightly hungry
5. No longer hungry but not yet satisfied
6. Comfortably satisfied
7. Starting to feel full
8. Feeling quite full
9. Starting to get a stomachache from so much food
10. In actual pain from overeating

The goal is for her to stay between a 3 and a 7 on the hunger scale. The next time she scores over 4 on the scale, have her drink an eight-ounce glass of water. It might take up to fifteen minutes for her hypothalamus (the region of the brain that functions as the main autonomic control center and regulates a person's appetite, among other things) to send a signal letting her nervous system know that her body was merely thirsty and that the thirst has been satisfied. If, after that time, she still feels hungry, then she can eat. She should never let herself get to a 1 or any other extreme.

Questions she should consider before she eats include[35]:

1. When was the last time she ate?
2. If it was less than two or three hours ago, she might not be feeling real hunger.
3. Could a small, nutritious snack rich in fiber tide her over until the next meal?
4. Can she drink a glass of water and wait twenty minutes?

It is also important for her to know the following differences among types of hunger and other sensations that may sometimes be confused with hunger, such as thirst, desire, and cravings. Inform her of the following differences:

PHYSICAL HUNGER: She experiences an empty sensation or hollowness in her stomach, which often comes with stomach rumblings, growling, and/or nausea. If it's ignored long enough, it can lead to low blood sugar and shakiness, weakness, and a light-headed feeling. These feelings don't come directly from her stomach, but rather from her blood glycogen levels and sometimes a depletion of vitamins and minerals.

EMOTIONAL HUNGER: It comes on suddenly because of an event (e.g., she is nervous or worried because she's in a play), experience (e.g., she had a misunderstanding with a friend), and/or an emotional trigger (e.g., she's feeling bored). She craves specific food(s) to comfort her.

DESIRE: Also referred to as mouth hunger,[36] this is eating for sheer flavor and a need for enjoyment. It drives people to seek out different tastes and textures in foods.

THIRST: She feels a dry sensation in her mouth, and she has a need to take in liquid.

CRAVINGS: She has a strong urge to eat a specific food, which comes with tension and an unpleasant yearning sensation in her mouth, throat, or body.

To illustrate how a craving is different from hunger, you could provide her with the following example: She has just eaten a meal but wants something specific, such as a cupcake, afterward. She might have been socialized into this ritual (having a sweet dessert following a meal) or learned it over time. She has a *desire* to eat a cupcake because she remembers how delicious it tasted the last time she ate one. After the meal she *craves* "only" a cupcake and doesn't want to settle for anything else. A bowl of strawberries, a banana, or anything else just won't satiate the craving. It is obviously not *hunger* that is causing her to gravitate toward the cupcake. If it was actual hunger, any food would do to satiate the hunger, as opposed to having it be "specifically" the cupcake.

Rating Your Hunger

Have your child monitor her hunger over the course of approximately three days. Try to have her do it both on days when she has a structured schedule and when she has free time (school days and the weekend). See if there is noticeable variation between those days. She can use the following chart to monitor her hunger.

RATING YOUR HUNGER
(0 BEING THE WEAKEST AND 5 THE STRONGEST)

TIME OF DAY (include specific time)	HOW I PHYSICALLY FEEL	STRENGTH OF HUNGER (0-5)	IS THIS DUE TO ACTUAL HUNGER, DESIRE, CRAVING, OR THIRST?
Before Breakfast:			
During Breakfast:			
Following Breakfast:			
Before Lunch:			
During Lunch:			
Following Lunch:			
Before Dinner:			
During Dinner:			
Following Dinner:			
Early Evening:			
Late Evening:			
Notes (What did you notice and learn about yourself?):			

WHEN THE MUNCHIES STRIKE

Assess Cravings

It's normal to have an urge or craving for certain types of food. We all have them! Cravings—a desire for a select food—may happen spontaneously or because we were triggered in some way. Whatever the reason, your child has the power to work through his craving. Everyone works through these urges differently. For some, giving in to cravings leads to unplanned and impulsive eating, while for others, having a small amount of that certain food is enough to ease the craving. If giving in to cravings leads your child to a place of overeating and carrying shameful feelings, the anti-craving strategies below can be helpful. You can review the following example, have him assess his cravings by filling out the chart, and go over the strategies with him.

CRAVING EXAMPLE: You just got home from school and had a snack on the way home to hold you over until dinner. You know that dinner is in about an hour. When you get home, you eye the leftover cake from celebrating your sister's birthday the night before. You can't get the picture out of your mind: the frosting, fluffy center, and how delicious it was. You remember eating more than your share the night before. You recognize you aren't particularly hungry and know that you'll be eating dinner soon, but the feelings are overwhelming. You decide to just have a little sliver to satisfy your craving. Before you know it, half the cake is finished, because you kept justifying just a little more, just a little more. However strange it seems, it literally felt as if the cake was talking directly to you and was trying to woo you. You are left feeling ashamed and disappointed that you gave in to the craving.

EXERCISE: Evaluating Your Cravings

Have your child evaluate his cravings so that he has greater awareness about the specific foods, time of day, level of discomfort, and what strategies are most effective to curb the cravings. With greater awareness, there's more of chance that mindful strategies will be used. Try to do it over a period of three days, during both structured (school days) and less structured days (on the weekend), to see if there's any variation.

EVALUATING CRAVINGS[37]

DAY AND TIME OF CRAVING			
How uncomfortable was the craving? (Scale of 0–5, 0 being the least, 5 the most.)			
How long did the craving last?			
What was going through my mind throughout the craving?			
Did I use any anti-craving techniques (drank water, listened to music, etc.)? If so, list them.			
Which techniques worked the best or didn't work at all?			

Thinking Techniques

Here are several mental techniques your child can try when faced with cravings:

- Assess whether it is in fact a craving and if it is centered on a specific food. (Signs include: your child's mind keeps gravitating toward thoughts of that food; he thinks, I must have it; and he wants it whether or not he's hungry or has recently eaten).
- Recognize that it's a craving. He should acknowledge that he is having a craving and self-talk to notice its presence at the moment. Once he brings it to his conscious awareness, this will slow him down and enable him to think through the process, as opposed to just acting out and giving in to the craving impulsively.
- Use imagery to imagine how he would think and feel if he were to give in to the craving and how he would think and feel if he were to successfully work through the challenge.
- Remind himself why he wants to empower himself and embrace his values and goals of healthful eating. Reinforce the belief that he has the capacity to work through the craving. By practicing being with his hunger and discomfort, he will build confidence and tolerance, which will make it easier for him to work through it in the future. Realize that by focusing on the present and looking at the bigger picture, he is actively working on empowering himself and building his self-acceptance and strengthening the belief that he can thrive in the midst of challenges.

Behavioral Techniques

If he is still tempted to give in to his cravings after engaging in self-talk, then encourage him to try as many of these behavioral techniques as he may need:

- Keep distance from the food he craves, particularly if the craving is especially strong and feels overpowering. He could even ask himself, on a scale from 1 (weakest) to 5 (strongest), how strong is his craving? This necessitates being honest with himself about the degree of his discomfort. Having access to the food when the craving is considerably strong can make it more difficult to resist the craving. If the food is around him because he's at a social function, he should walk away from being in direct contact with it or ask that it be removed from where he is. He could work on building tolerance progressively when his craving is manageable and when he's in a more structured setting. Inevitably, his goal is to be directly exposed to the discomfort and make mindful, positive decisions while accepting the discomfort.

- Find alternative ways to cope with the oral fixation and/or desire to eat. Drink water, eat a healthier food or snack, etc.
- Engage in stress management and relaxation techniques (such as deep breathing, meditation, yoga).
- If the craving is at an extremely high level of intensity, de-escalate the situation with the items on the next list. He can gauge each item's effectiveness based on its ability to help him through the craving.

EXERCISE: Activities to De-escalate Cravings

In addition to the thinking and behavioral techniques described, ask your child to try using these activities when cravings are at an all-time peak and the intensity of feelings doesn't allow for other mindfulness or problem-solving techniques.

Assess how effective these activities are (or think back to a time when you tried to distract yourself from a craving. Rate the effectiveness of these activities to suppress cravings on a scale from 0 (not effective at all) to 5 (most effective).

DISTRACTION LIST	EFFECTIVENESS
❏ Write in a journal	_____
❏ Formulate and read power cards (see Chapter 4)	_____
❏ Surf the Internet	_____
❏ Write emails	_____
❏ Speak to a friend	_____

DISTRACTION LIST	EFFECTIVENESS
❏ Speak to a family member	_____
❏ Do mindfulness or stress management techniques	_____
❏ Watch television	_____
❏ Play a computer game	_____
❏ Play a board game/cards	_____
❏ Read a book or magazine	_____
❏ Do a puzzle/word game	_____
❏ Draw or do an arts and crafts project	_____
❏ Listen to music	_____
❏ Download new music	_____
❏ Play a musical instrument	_____
❏ Organize your room or something else	_____
❏ Play with a pet	_____
❏ Take a bike ride/walk/jog	_____
❏ Brush your teeth	_____
❏ Take a bath/shower	_____
❏ Polish your nails	_____
❏ Chew gum	_____
❏ Drink water or a low-calorie beverage	_____
❏ Other _____	_____
❏ Other _____	_____
❏ Other _____	_____

Keep in mind that your child's initial feeling may often be "I can't stand this," "I must have it," "This is too hard," and "I can't be without it." Through consistent and persistent practice, he will recognize that he *can* stand his craving, he can effectively work through it, and that it is hard at times but not impossible. *Cravings eventually pass, and we shouldn't react to them quickly and mindlessly.*

GIVING IN TO THE CRAVING

Sometimes your child may give in to the craving if the urge is especially strong and lingering. Seek to help him put things into perspective, acknowledge his progress, and communicate that not all is lost. Support him by helping him understand what was difficult about that time (he can fill out the evaluation of a challenging situation in Chapter 11) so he can learn from it and "get back on the horse." Embracing the value of health is an ongoing process with challenging times and seamless ones—but it is part of a practice that he has courageously dedicated himself to.

There is also a distinction between giving in to one craving and sabotaging his overall goals by spiraling out of control—completely giving up on himself and his healthful eating and exercise behaviors. He has the power to recalibrate himself and gain awareness even while the craving behavior is actively in progress. At any point, he can choose to become more mindful and behave in a value-driven way. The power is in his hands!

STRATEGY 17

HALT

Learn About Emotional Eating

It is common for kids and teens to use food as a coping mechanism for dealing with overwhelming emotions. Food is easily accessible and reliable. Many kids and teens in my focus groups reported that they have used food to comfort them from loneliness and boredom and have also learned to use food to reinforce positive emotions, such as when they socialize or attend celebratory occasions. They acknowledged the major role of food embedded in many celebrations and holidays that is ingrained in the fabric of our culture.

Emotional eating can be influenced by both positive and negative emotions. Feelings can affect a child's motivation to eat, her food choices, where and with whom she eats, and how quickly she eats a meal.[38] This can be conscious or unconscious behavior.

The cycle of emotional eating includes a situation ➜ an intense emotion ➜ eating to avoid or soothe.[39] This leads to negative emotions (e.g., sadness, nervousness) that drive her to overeat ➜ her emotions return often with an additional burden of guilt because she overate and compromised her healthful values and goals only to feel increasingly worse (ashamed and guilty that she overate) ➜ unhealthy and frustrating cycle gets perpetuated over time. It's no wonder that a kid or teen would want to avoid an uncomfortable emotion. In Chapter 1, when we discussed mindfulness, you learned how our mind naturally copes with these.

If your child emotionally eats, she may not be paying attention to her body. Rather than satisfying hunger, she may be reacting to an emotion such as boredom, anxiety, or loneliness. When that happens, "eating becomes disconnected from nourishment and instead becomes an automatic reaction to negative emotions, misunderstood physical sensations, and mental stress that has little to do with being hungry."[40] Once that learned behavior is in place, your child needs to relearn how to react to her emotions and get in touch with her body's hunger cues and craving sensations.

To understand the emotions behind why she is eating, she can take note of the acronym HALT: **H**appy, **A**ngry/**A**nxious, **L**onely, or **T**ired. Other common reasons kids overeat are boredom and/or frustration. Comfort foods are often consumed to soothe a bad mood (loneliness) or to stay in a good mood (when celebrating). Typical comfort foods include ice cream, chocolate, pizza, chips, steak, and peanut butter.

A study on comfort foods found that the types people are drawn to vary depending on their moods. People in happy moods tend to prefer foods such as pizza and steak (32 percent). Sad people reach for ice cream and cookies (39 percent), and bored people open up a bag of potato chips (36 percent). The most important finding, however, is that both gender and age influence one's preference of comfort foods. Females tend to prefer snack-related comfort foods, while males prefer more meal-related foods. In addition, younger people prefer snack-related foods when compared to older people.[41]

It is evident that emotional eating can get in the way of your child carrying out her healthful eating and exercise behaviors. It is important that your child becomes aware of the difference between emotional hunger and physical hunger to avoid overeating as a result of emotional triggers. You can convey to her the differences, why she may be turning to food for emotional reasons, what triggers she may observe, and how she can avoid emotional eating behaviors that thwart her healthful values and goals.

DIFFERENTIATING BETWEEN EMOTIONAL HUNGER AND PHYSICAL HUNGER

1. Emotional hunger comes on very suddenly and is urgent, whereas physical hunger comes on slowly and can be postponed.

66

2. With emotional hunger, your child craves a specific food, and only that food will meet her need. With physical hunger, the need can be satisfied by a number of different foods.

3. With emotional hunger, even when she's full, she is more likely to continue eating because she's attempting to satisfy an emotional need. With physical hunger, she's more likely to stop eating when she's feeling full.

4. Emotional eating often leaves behind feelings of guilt and shame because of the impulsivity compelling the behavior—eating when she's physically hungry does not evoke feelings of guilt. Once the hunger is satisfied, the eating ceases.

Emotional reasons your child may turn to food:

1. She experienced a stressful event or experience.

2. She is feeling scared and/or anxious.

3. She is feeling sad.

4. She is feeling unbelievably happy.

Be aware and HALT (**H**appy, **A**ngry/**A**nxious, **L**onely, or **T**ired) in the midst of emotional eating.

Engaging in emotional eating is often a way to keep feelings blocked, locked, or buried. Common triggers are daily life stressors (usual things that come up, such as schoolwork, socializing with friends, etc.), a major life event (a birthday, graduation, etc.), or a trauma (a reminder of something bad that happened to her). Examples of triggers include:

- Feeling sad because she had a challenging day at school (emotional)
- Feeling disappointed because of an argument with a friend (social)
- Feeling tired/exhausted (physiological)
- Seeing an advertisement for food (situational)
- Thinking about how she'll "never" be able to carry out healthful behaviors (thinking)

According to dietitian Jane Jakubczak, 75 percent of overeating is caused by emotions. She expressed that this is why we need to learn techniques besides eating that help us manage our emotions. "Oftentimes when a child is sad, we cheer them up with a sweet treat. This behavior gets reinforced year after year until we are practicing the same behavior as adults. We never learn to deal with the sad feeling because we push it away with a sweet treat. Learning to deal with feelings without food is a new skill many of us need to learn."[42]

To avoid emotional eating, have your child do the following:

1. Observe yourself and complete an emotional-eating record (see page 69) over the course of three days, including both structured and unstructured days. This way, you can become aware of the events or triggers that compel the eating and how you might otherwise act in those situations.

2. Use the 4Ps strategy—predict (how you will behave), plan (what you will do about it), put the plan into action, and continually practice (the 4Ps will be explained more in depth in Chapter 5).

3. Slow down and create space for thoughtful problem solving. Pause and take eight seconds before you act.

4. Use mindfulness, stress management, and self-soothing techniques (e.g., exercise, listening to music, talking with a parent or friend).

5. Get support and comfort for the underlying emotions (sadness, frustration, anger). Seek help from a support group, psychotherapist, family, or peers.

6. Take away overly intense temptations by initially distracting yourself; then use mindfulness strategies to be present with your emotion.

7. Get enough sleep. Tiredness can sometimes feel like hunger.

8. Cherish yourself and learn to self-soothe in more nurturing ways (e.g., read, take a nature walk, play with a pet).

9. Comfort foods don't need to be unhealthy. Identify healthy alternative foods that can serve as a comfort food for you.

EXERCISE: Record Your Emotional Eating Situations

Ask your child to think back to the time she last engaged in emotional eating. Have her fill out the following chart and record the situation, event, or trigger, what thoughts and feelings arose, and what action she took or plans on taking in the future.

EMOTIONAL EATING RECORD

EVENT OR SITUATION/ TRIGGER	THOUGHTS	FEELINGS	DIRECT ACTION TAKEN OR TO TAKE
Example: I got into an argument with my mother.	I deserve and will make myself feel better by eating ice cream and chocolate.	I am feeling hopeless, sad, and frustrated.	I chatted with a supportive friend where I was able to share my feelings, and later I listened to my favorite music and tapped into my sadness.

A situation, event, or trigger may cause uncomfortable feelings that can directly impact your child's behavior. Habitually she may overeat to avoid confronting those feelings. Having an awareness of this cycle and knowledge about alternative coping strategies can help her make more mindful decisions.

STRATEGY 18

EAT WITH INTENTION

Use Intuitive and Mindful Eating Practices

Establishing healthy eating habits is a much more effective approach for kids than dieting (this will be further explored in Chapter 5), restricting foods, and/or micromanaging their portion sizes. Researchers found that restricting children can work in the short term, but in the long term it can increase food intake and eating in the absence of hunger, hamper children's ability to self-regulate, cause negative self-evaluation, and contribute to weight gain.[43]

To date, more than twenty-five studies show that intuitive eaters, rather than emotional ones, have lower body mass index levels and fewer eating disorders, eat a variety of foods, enjoy eating, have better cholesterol levels, and possess a psychological hardiness, which includes well-being and resilience.[44]

Intuitive eaters hold the belief that no diet or meal plan could possibly "get" your child's hunger and fullness levels or what truly satisfies him. Only he knows his thoughts, feelings, and experiences. He's the ultimate expert on himself.

It is not possible to sequester kids from any type of situation in which they are exposed to food, nor do we want to. It will always be around, and they will always be tempted. Who isn't? The objective is to teach kids skills so that they learn to make good, balanced decisions about their eating behavior independently, intuitively, and mindfully. Here are some ways to do so:

- Convey to your child that no foods are off-limits or are labeled as "bad" or "good," "healthy" or "unhealthy," "junk," etc. You can refer to one food over another as a healthier choice while still empowering your child to make that choice.
- Let him know all foods are permissible if eaten mindfully and in moderation.

70

- If there are certain foods that instantly trigger overeating behavior, these select foods may initially need to be curtailed. Introduce this process as an experiment rather than a punishment, and only follow through with it if your child is fully on board with the plan to prevent his obsessing over and seeking out those foods, whether in secret or in the open.
- Foster self-regulation by helping your child get in touch with his natural eating habits. Get kids in tune with when they are physically hungry and satisfied, and the differences among hunger, desire, thirst, and cravings.
- Encourage him to not skip meals or healthful snacks. This can lead to mindless or impulsive eating because of being overly hungry or feeling deprived.
- Have him practice leaving food on his plate as opposed to finishing every morsel. A valuable skill is learning to sit with discomfort, as opposed to avoiding or getting rid of his feelings. This will help him when he inevitably experiences cravings.
- Help him get in touch with his hunger cues; for example, start with small servings and portions, and let your child ask for more if he is still hungry.
- Foster independent thinking and decision making by teaching him about healthy portion sizes and what they look like (see serving size chart on page 72). Do not micromanage and criticize him if he digresses from the standard. He inevitably has to decide for himself. (For younger kids, ages ten to thirteen, provide more direct guidance, and for teens fourteen to eighteen, less direct guidance.)
- Teach him to savor food and eat slowly so that he is not on autopilot. Rather than mindlessly gobbling or swallowing, he is intentionally paying attention to aromas, texture, consistency, and taste.
- Be open to your child having access to foods when he is physically hungry rather than only during structured mealtimes. Kids and teens have higher rates of metabolism than adults because of their developmental growth spurts, and they may need different eating schedules than you do.
- Provide a variety of healthier foods to choose from.
- Based on the mindfulness eating cycle, help your child notice his direct experiences by assessing *why* he is eating, *where* he is eating

(where he's investing energy), *when* he wants to eat, *how* much he wants to eat, *what* he wants to eat, and *in what way* (mindfully).[45]

SERVING SIZE CHART[46]

BASIC GUIDELINES	GRAINS	DAIRY, FATS, AND OILS
1 cup = baseball	1 cup of cereal flakes = baseball	1½ oz cheese = 3 stacked dice
½ cup = lightbulb	1 pancake = DVD	1 cup yogurt = baseball
1 oz or 2 tbsp = golf ball	½ cup cooked rice = lightbulb	½ cup frozen yogurt = lightbulb
1 tbsp = poker chip	½ cup cooked pasta = lightbulb	½ cup ice cream = lightbulb
3 oz meat = deck of cards	1 slice bread = smartphone	1 tbsp butter or spread = poker chip
3 oz fish = smartphone	1 bagel = 6 oz can of tuna	1 tbsp salad dressing = poker chip
	3 cups popcorn = 3 baseballs	1 tbsp oil = poker chip
		1 tbsp mayonnaise = poker chip
FRUITS AND VEGETABLES	**MEATS, FISH, AND NUTS**	**MIXED DISHES**
1 medium fruit = baseball	3 oz lean meat = deck of cards	1 hamburger (without bun) = deck of cards
½ cup grapes = about 16 grapes	3 oz fish = smartphone	1 cup fries = about 10 fries
1 cup strawberries = about 12 berries	3 oz tofu = deck of cards	4 oz nachos = about 7 chips
1 cup salad greens = baseball	2 tbsp peanut butter = golf ball	3 oz meatloaf = deck of cards
1 cup carrots = about 12 baby carrots	2 tbsp hummus = golf ball	1 cup chili = baseball
1 cup cooked vegetables = baseball	¼ cup almonds = 23 almonds	1 sub sandwich = about 6 inches
1 baked potato = computer mouse	¼ cup pistachios = 24 pistachios	1 burrito = about 6 inches

*For a kid- and teen-friendly quiz about serving sizes, visit rd.com/slideshows/ portion-distortion-serving-sizes.

FREE YOUR CHILD FROM OVEREATING

We all sometimes become distracted when we eat. With distractions we often don't recognize how much food we're consuming. *Find ways to focus on the foods that you are eating.* Some mindful ways to accomplish this include:

EAT SLOWLY: Appreciate every bite. Practicing this means being aware of all tastes, aromas, textures, and consistencies and pausing in between bites and during transitions between courses. Pause during the meal by putting down your utensils during bites. Practice this at home, when eating out, and at school. The more you notice and appreciate the food you eat, the more satisfied you will feel.

Eating slowly is also beneficial because it gives you the opportunity to become full before consuming more than you intended or nutritionally needed. It usually takes 20 minutes to feel physically full. Eating slowly gives the brain time to receive signals from digestive hormones secreted by the gastrointestinal tract. Research suggests that the hormone leptin also interacts with the neurotransmitter dopamine in the brain to produce a feeling of pleasure after eating. The theory is that, by eating too quickly, people may not give this intricate hormonal system enough time to work.[47] If you're shoveling food in, you're typically not giving yourself enough time to register that you're satiated and to appreciate all that you're eating.

EAT IN A SETTING THAT ENHANCES CONCENTRATION AND FOCUS ON YOUR FOOD: When eating, attempt to be in a setting that is relatively quiet and stress-free. This will allow you to focus on your food and appreciate its temperature, texture, and flavors. Close your eyes to take in the different tastes. It is helpful to set the standard that food is to be eaten in places such as the kitchen or at the table. Food that is eaten in other areas, such as the family room or in a car, tends to be eaten in haste.

BE AWARE OF AND ELIMINATE DISTRACTIONS: We are all distracted by outside stimuli such as the TV, computers, video games, phones, etc. In order to facilitate mindful practice, it is essential to keep these down to a minimum when eating. Follow the general rule that mealtimes are spent distraction-free—no smartphones, movies, TV, etc.

SIT DOWN WHEN EATING: Whenever possible, sit down while you eat. Because of our overscheduled lives, we often find ourselves standing and eating. This happens haphazardly when we're eating "out of the refrigerator" or "on the go." There may be times when you opt for less healthy choices because you're eating on the run.

CONSIDER SERVING SIZE: Whether it's a meal or snack, to ensure proper nutrition, it is helpful to learn appropriate portion sizes. Awareness and education about portion control is known to be a major issue contributing to the effectiveness of weight and health management.[48] It's no fault of kids and teens that "supersize" portions are the norm in restaurants in the United States. Kids and teens are used to observing the glorification of larger portions.

You might portion out everything prior to a meal and put the containers with the leftover amount back in the refrigerator. If you are cooking or are having the food cooked for you, portion out the amount that you will eat and put the rest away. Typically, extra servings are at the table, which can lead to overeating and double and triple portion sizes. Keeping the extra food out of sight enforces mindful planning and practice.

Create your own snack packs with snack-size, resealable bags. If you reach into a full bag, you are likely to grab more than you intended. *Snacking can be addicting.* Because snacking on something sweet, salty, or crunchy is pleasurable, it stimulates the brain's reward centers through the neurotransmitter dopamine, exactly like other addictive drugs, and releases the body's own opioids in the brain, sending signals that it needs more.[49] You can't help but want more. Your body is just naturally reacting! Planning ahead is the best strategy to combat over-snacking.

EXERCISE: Mindful Eating

Have your child do this exercise as he is sitting down at the table to eat lunch or dinner. Ask him to mindfully commit to eating slowly and without distractions. Have him earmark at least thirty minutes for the meal and purposefully take pauses between bites and between courses if he is having several. During each bite, have him concentrate on what he is eating—every taste, aroma, texture, consistency—he should note them all. He should pay attention to the changes in the food, how his body reacts to the food, and whether he feels more or less full or satiated. Have him continue to eat slowly throughout, focusing on the food and his body and appreciating the sustenance he is getting.

After the meal, process the experience with him by asking:

- What was it like eating slowly?
- What was it like eating without distractions?
- What was it like taking pauses in between bites and different courses?
- What did you notice about your thoughts through the process?
- What did you notice in your body through the process?

By engaging in mindful eating practices, he will eat with more intention. This enhances his decision making and gets him in tune with his thoughts, feelings, and the actions he takes in regard to his value of healthful eating.

CHECK YOUR BAGGAGE

As your child takes inventory of willingness, eating behaviors, hunger, cravings, and emotional eating, you may find out things that you didn't know or expect. Some of these things may evoke intense feelings for you, your child, or both of you. Be sure you process these feelings so that they don't spill over when you interact.

We often choose to see children a certain way or wish that they didn't have to face certain challenges. With the support and care of parents, kids and teens are more likely to invest in their health and be open to change. You can also help work through your child's own personal feelings. Part of the process is for your child to be more self-aware and gain self-acceptance. Your unconditional love can help facilitate the process and decrease feelings of shame, hopelessness, or any other emotions that may arise.

Your child is also learning to evaluate emotional eating. Researchers have found that "higher levels of emotional eating by parents were related to higher levels of adolescents' emotional eating."[50] As a parent, it's critical to take an inventory of your own eating behaviors and note their potential impact on your child. You are responsible for modeling appropriate healthful behaviors so that your child has the benefit of positive examples. Kids and teens are attuned to when parents don't "practice what they preach." They are more likely to resist change and have a challenging time justifying why they should put in the effort.

You want to be sure to model eating with intention as well as eating mindfully and thoughtfully. The exercises in this chapter challenged your child to think and act differently than your child is probably used to. When kids and teens are challenged to push their limits, they may feel awkward, resist, or be suspicious and cautious. Allow them to think how they think and feel how they feel, and try to reserve judgment. Allow them to explain their point of view and express their reluctance (or excitement). Hear them out fully, and be open to a dialogue about their concerns. As you support them through the process, reinforce that they are entitled to see things their way and that you are there to listen and continue on this journey with them.

 ## REVIEW

You committed to extensive self-exploration in this chapter, had the opportunity to assess willingness to change, eating behaviors, hunger, cravings, and emotional eating. You now understand the differences among physical hunger, emotional hunger, desire, thirst, and cravings. Additionally, you have learned specific strategies to de-escalate cravings. You have explored emotional eating and ways to avoid it. Finally, you had the opportunity to learn about mindfulness-based eating and how to eat with intention and self-awareness. You have gained awareness of your health and acquired mindfulness-based eating behaviors.

Kids and teens learned about:

- Willingness to invest in the practice of healthy eating
- Hunger and cravings
- How to HALT emotional eating
- Types of hunger
- Serving sizes
- Mindfulness-based eating.

 ## MINDFULNESS EXERCISE: Your Journey

See page 220 for the mindfulness exercise that corresponds to this chapter, and refer to page 217 for instructions on accessing the audio.

4

It's All in the Mind

I always go for doubles and triples [servings] when I'm at a party and there's a buffet. I can't help it. Something comes over me, and I say to myself, "I just have to have it." Then I ask myself, "When is the next time I'll have this?" I'm left feeling annoyed at myself and say, "I won't do this again." I know this is bullshit, but I always buy into it.

—SHARON, AGE 17

When I'm with my friends at school, I feel so much pressure. They're all snacking, and I don't want to stand out as the only one who has to watch her weight. They'll notice I'm not eating what they're eating and think I'm fat.

—REBECCA, AGE 13

THOUGHTS AND FEELINGS CAN BE unpredictable. They're influenced by our past experiences, our hormones, how much sleep we got, and how confident we're feeling in general. This is true for everyone. It's important to help your child realize we can't control our thoughts and feelings, only the actions we choose to take. Using the techniques in this chapter, you can help your child acquire flexibility in order to make thoughtful decisions no matter what thoughts and feelings come up.

As an example, your child may have strong cravings for a third cookie at a party. Even though it is clear that she is experiencing a craving, she may be thinking that she "shouldn't" have this craving. Because she wants the cookie anyway, she concludes that she "can't control herself" and has no willpower. She gives up on trying to work through the craving because of the thought: "What's the point? I can't control myself now and never will be able to." She eats the cookie and is left feeling guilty and ashamed.

Knowing and accepting themselves will empower kids and teens to work more effectively with what comes their way, as opposed to wanting to get rid of parts of themselves. This cycle of negativity leads to negative sentiments—shame, personal disapproval, resentment, and eventually self-hatred. It chips away at a child's self-confidence, self-worth, and self-compassion. It's a cycle we want to avoid! Kids and teens will be less likely to invest in trying to make a change if they don't have confidence in themselves, feel they have value, and believe that they can effectively pursue a meaningful life.

STRATEGY 19

TRIGGER ID-ING

Understand Triggers

Thinking tends to start with a trigger, something that makes us want to act. When triggers block more complex thinking, we react quickly and impulsively. We rationalize (create explanations or excuses for) our behavior to justify it to ourselves or others (see Strategy 21). Here's the way it may appear for your child:

TRIGGER CYCLE

SHE GETS TRIGGERED.	Someone offers her a third slice of pizza.
⬇	
SHE EXPERIENCES A THOUGHT.	"The pizza looks good." "It smells so good." "The last one was so tasty." "I want it."
⬇	
SHE RATIONALIZES.	"I deserve it because I had a challenging day." "It will help me feel better." "I usually don't have three slices." "It will be just this once." "I will eat less tomorrow."
⬇	
SHE ACTS.	She eats the third slice of pizza even though she feels slightly full. She hasn't waited the twenty minutes for her brain to recognize and report back to her whether physically she was in fact feeling full or not.
⬇	
AFTER SHE ACTS, SHE THINKS:	"Why can't I control myself? I'm so weak and out of control." "I am really annoyed with myself because I did not want or need that third slice of pizza." "What's the point of trying? I might as well accept that I'm bad at this and not much is going to change."
⬇	
SHE FEELS:	Angry, frustrated, sad, and hopeless.

Examples of triggers include:

- Feeling down after not being invited to a party (emotional)
- A misunderstanding with a loved one or friend (social)
- Feeling ill (physiological)
- Attending a wedding (situational)
- Thinking about how things "should" or "shouldn't be" (thinking)

EXERCISE: Identify Your Triggers

Collaborate with your child to identify if her triggers are on all five levels. Chart her triggers, thoughts, rationalizations, actions, and her thinking after she acts.

EMOTIONAL TRIGGERS: _____

SOCIAL TRIGGERS: _____

PHYSIOLOGICAL TRIGGERS: _____

SITUATIONAL TRIGGERS: _____

THINKING: _____

If you help your child get to know herself better, she'll gain an understanding about what triggers her to engage in unplanned eating, overeating, and unhealthful choices. She will get more in tune with herself and conscientious when she is taking action.

For example, your child identifies a trigger situation: when the Girl Scouts come around selling cookies. In the past, she told herself she would just stop at eating two Girl Scout cookies, but this rarely sticks, and she typically ends up eating half the box. She recognizes that there is good reason to believe that it can happen again if she doesn't plan in advance. Her plan may include portioning out the cookies, eating two and throwing the rest out (better to be wasted in the garbage than wasted in her body), or giving the rest away. She learns to consult with family members about what works best for them and thinks about her own needs.

Most kids and teens don't think before they act and go from trigger to action before they realize it. Though this is partially due to where they are developmentally, kids and teens still have a great capacity to learn about their thoughts and feelings and to make changes in their behavior. *By understanding her triggers, instead of acting on impulse, your child gains the chance to act by choice.*

STRATEGY 20

RETHINK STINKING THINKING

Identify Self-Sabotaging Thought Patterns

Your goal for your child should not be to change his thoughts but to help him observe them, study them, and choose a mindful action in response. If he believes everything he thinks and never evaluates it, inevitably he'll come upon situations in which he perceives things differently from how they actually are. These perceptions—which Dr. Aaron Beck, founder of Cognitive-Behavioral Therapy, terms "cognitive distortions" or "thinking errors"—can get in the way of achieving goals and acting on behalf of personal values.[51] My term for this is "stinking thinking."

Just like positive thinking, stinking thinking sets in motion the way your child experiences a situation or circumstance, the way he thinks and feels about it, and then the way he acts. For example, if a high school student participates in but loses his playoff baseball game, he may understandably feel frustrated. He might have a hard time getting past the feeling. He thinks, "What was the point of playing the whole season? We lost the playoff game and are out of the running." He may convince himself, "The coach is disappointed in us and thinks we suck." Since this thinking makes him feel sad and ashamed, he may neglect to thank his coach for guidance throughout the season or appreciate his teammates' efforts. He may even want to skip the awards dinner and decide he doesn't want to try out for the next season.

In thinking this way, he's "minimizing" the effort he and his team put in. Okay, parts of the season were weak, but his team still made it to the playoffs because they won games and played well. And his guesses about his coach's opinion of him are another kind of stinking thinking, known as "mind reading."

Stinking thinking takes many forms. In this situation, it led our baseball player to want to quit the team after one bad game. Quitting would cause him to lose out on a source of physical fitness. There are many other situations in which stinking thinking can affect healthy eating and exercise behaviors. It can sabotage your child's motivation, making it less

80

likely that he will stick with the practice; that's why it is essential to understand how it works and how to work through it.

THE MOST COMMON TYPES OF STINKING THINKING[52]

1. **ALL-OR-NOTHING THINKING:** Black-and-white thinking with nothing in the middle

   Taylor has eaten healthily all week. At lunch on Saturday, she eats a healthy sub and feels content. Later, her friends want to get an ice-cream sundae. She goes along with the group and has a three-scoop hot fudge sundae. Guilt creeps in after she finishes. She tells herself, "I've blown my healthy eating plan. I might as well go off it for the rest of the weekend and start fresh next Monday."

   Taylor's all-or-nothing thinking keeps her from recognizing that one sundae is not the end of the world and that totally giving up for a weekend is not in line with her goals. If anything, it will only pull her away from accomplishing what she wants. She could consider that she can have the sundae *and* stay with her plan—maybe even make a dent in the sundae calories by walking to school for the upcoming week instead of riding the bus.

2. **CATASTROPHIZING:** Negative fortune-telling

   Nate followed his healthy eating plan all week, exercised regularly by participating in intramurals, and felt aware of his triggers. But as he zips up his jeans, he can tell that he hasn't lost any weight. He thinks, "I'm doomed. I'll never slim down for baseball season." He binges on three cupcakes.

   If he had not had these catastrophic thoughts, he might contemplate other explanations for not losing weight this week. Perhaps it's water weight or a weight-loss plateau. He could reconsider by reminding himself that eating healthily is a process and a practice. The end result will be better health even if he hasn't lost weight this week.

3. **EMOTIONAL REASONING:** Thinking your ideas must be true even though evidence says otherwise

   Shay has been on track, eating healthily and exercising, and her weight has been inching down. She argues with her best friend and feels really sad about it. "Time to hit the snack drawer," she

81

IT'S ALL IN THE MIND

tells herself. "A couple of candy bars always makes me feel better." After Shay comes off the sugar buzz, she's still sad, and on top of it, she's disappointed in herself, too.

To reconsider, Shay could find ways to cope other than emotional eating. She might walk to clear her mind, listen to her favorite music to gain perspective, or call her friend to work it out.

4. **MAGNIFICATION/MINIMIZATION**: Making the negative bigger and the positive smaller

Troy did a great job all week mindfully adding vegetables and fruits to his food plan. On Friday, he didn't include either one and ate past feeling full. "I'm worthless and have no willpower," he tells himself.

If Troy were not engaged in magnified thinking, he might reconsider and say, "Even though I didn't include a fruit or vegetable, even though I ate a little more than I meant to, I've made great choices lately." Troy would then be proud of himself and feel confident that he can continue to be successful and put meaningful effort toward the practice. By reconsidering and thinking positively, Troy will feel motivated to stay on track.

Troy also doesn't want to minimize the situation. When he doesn't hold himself accountable, saying it's no big deal can lead him to participate in undesirable behavior again. Instead, Troy can learn from his unintentional eating, for the future. Troy realizes if he continues to practice, he'll have fewer of these moments, resulting in improved health.

5. **MENTAL FILTER**: Paying undue attention to one negative detail of the situation instead of seeing the whole picture

Haden stayed up late to finish his part in a group project. In the morning, he doesn't hear the early alarm that would have allowed him to exercise on the track before school. There's no other time to fit it in. Haden thinks, "I can't exercise today, which means I'm not doing anything productive toward my health."

If he expanded his thinking, he would reconsider and recognize that he was productive in other ways. He completed his project, and jogging the track is not the only form of exercise he gets each day. He climbs up and down the stairs at school or work, participates in a football game, and walks the dog. All of these count as cardiovascular exercise!

6. **MIND READING:** Believing you know what others are thinking

Nina is at a restaurant that does not have a "lighter" menu, but she wants to eliminate the creamed salad dressing and croutons from her salad. She glances up from her menu and tells herself, "I want to make this request, but I can tell from the waiter's expression, he'll be annoyed and tell me it's impossible to make changes to the food order."

If Nina reconsidered reading the mind of the waiter, she would be more inclined to make her requests. Nina would remind herself that part of the waiter's job is to help her get the meal she wants and needs. Plus, Nina isn't making extraordinary or difficult demands. If she had an allergy, she wouldn't hesitate to ask for what she needed. It is within her rights to ask in a respectful way for accommodations for her health needs. Lastly, she would acknowledge that these days many people are trying to improve their health, and the waiter is probably accustomed to being asked.

7. **SELF-DELUDING THINKING:** Rationalizing by telling yourself things you do not really believe

At dinner, Emma resists taking seconds, which she really wanted. Her father congratulates her on her achievement. That night she sneaks down and raids the refrigerator. "If my parents can't see me eating, it doesn't really count," she tells herself.

If Emma were not engaged in self-deluding thinking, she would know that her behavior still counts, even though no one is watching her, and that it doesn't reflect her integrity or support her goals. Rather than raid the refrigerator for high-calorie, sugary foods, she might grab an apple and go back to her room.

8. **UNHELPFUL RULES:** Making decisions without taking circumstances into consideration

All the sugary snacks in Megan's house pose a major challenge for her. They sit in the cabinet within easy reach, tempting her. She decides she cannot ask her family to be supportive and vary or limit the snacks. Megan is following the "rule" that it is not right to impose on others who do not have difficulty with overindulging. "If I say something, they'll think I'm inconsiderate; I'll make them uncomfortable," she tells herself. Because of this rule, she remains silent, continues to have a difficult time fighting the temptations, and continues to overindulge.

83

If Megan were not obeying this unhelpful rule, she might consider that her family wants to be supportive and do whatever it takes to help her. Their help would come with warmth, pride, and acceptance and would make her feel comforted as she works toward these goals. She might also consider that they might appreciate the change because it could serve as a benefit to them, too.

9. **JUSTIFICATION:** Linking two unrelated concepts to justify your feelings

Cami is following her nutritionist's suggestion for snacks and eating unlimited servings of fresh fruit and vegetables. She just finished a well-balanced lunch and is feeling physically satiated, but a great-looking bowl of cherries tempts her. She decides to eat it even though she's not hungry and she's already had two servings of fruit today. "This is healthy. Eating fruit at any moment of the day, even after a full meal, is okay," she tells herself.

If Cami were not justifying her behavior, she might reconsider that, even though all fruit is nutritious, she's not hungry. She would acknowledge that even healthful fruit contains sugar and calories that she needs to consider. She could reconsider and wait to have it for a snack an hour before dinner, because that is when she typically gets hungry and eats a snack to hold her over.

10. **"SHOULD," "OUGHT TO," AND "MUST" STATEMENTS:** Insistence that things "should," "ought to," and "must" be as you like

Kim strongly believes that maintaining good health ought to be easy. Maintaining health should take little or no effort. She decides that if frustration or disappointments get in the way, then it is okay for her to quit, because being healthy must be easy.

If her thinking were more flexible and less rigid, Kim would reconsider and acknowledge that most things she wants to do well in life require effort and include some disappointment and frustration along the way. She would recognize that having some better days and some more challenging days is a natural part of the process. It won't be all bad or all good. Kim would recognize that difficult days don't stay forever—even though in the moment it may feel that way—and that she can get through them.

Learning about the stinking thinking that gets in the way of weight management will give you and your child specific patterns to look out for, as well as actions to take that combat cognitive distortions. To effectively help your child work through stinking thinking, you can:

1. Identify which forms pertain to your child;

2. Ask him if he can relate to the example that was provided. If so, ask him what aspects of it pertained to him, and if not, ask him to give you a personal example that relates directly to him;

3. Role-play with him based on the example given or on the one he provided. If he doesn't feel comfortable role-playing, just talk the scenario out or read it aloud.

4. Process with him his thoughts and feelings about being in that role, what challenges he thinks may come up for him, and how he will effectively work through them.

Throughout this process, be sure to let your child fully express himself. Be aware of your own feelings and reactions. Use active listening skills by not talking too much, probing, interrupting, or offering advice or solutions prematurely. Throughout the discussion, ask open-ended questions and convey warmth and support in regard to how he is thinking and feeling. (For more information on active listening skills, go to Chapter 7 on communication).

STRATEGY 21

~~1,001~~ ZERO EXCUSES

Recognize Common Rationalizations

We constantly rationalize our behavior. Unfortunately, when we justify behavior that we would rather not be doing or that is not especially helpful, we end up trying to control the feelings of shame, guilt, and frustration that soon follow. And we usually lose out. We recognize that we're making up excuses, and we're left with the self-disparaging thoughts and feelings that take up space.

Your child most likely engages in rationalizing when she eats foods she did not intend to, eats more than she planned, or doesn't stick to a plan she made for herself. In the list below, you'll see many common rationalizations. You may recognize some of them from your own thoughts, and others may seem right from the mouth of your child. She may repeat the same ones over and over again, or her rationalizations may change. Your child may also experience two or more of these excuses operating at once. Our thoughts and minds are fascinating (and fickle)!

EXERCISE: Common Rationalizations/Excuses[53]

Sit down with your child and have her check off each item on the list below that applies to her.

- ❏ Watching what I eat is too hard.
- ❏ It is not that fattening.
- ❏ I don't care.
- ❏ I will make up for it later.
- ❏ It is okay to eat this.
- ❏ It will go to waste if I don't eat it.
- ❏ I should eat it because it's free.
- ❏ It is not fair.
- ❏ Everyone else is eating.
- ❏ I am not going to let anyone tell me what I can or cannot eat.
- ❏ I don't want to disappoint or inconvenience _____.
- ❏ I deserve to eat this.
- ❏ I am anxious.
- ❏ I am tired.
- ❏ I am sad/upset.
- ❏ I am bored.
- ❏ I just exercised (played ball, ran, etc.), so I can have this.
- ❏ I will just eat these few nibbles.
- ❏ It is a special occasion.
- ❏ I am treating myself.
- ❏ I can start eating more healthfully again tomorrow.
- ❏ I really want it.
- ❏ I will never stick with this practice, anyway.
- ❏ It's freshly cooked/baked.
- ❏ No one will know.
- ❏ I have no willpower.
- ❏ I will end up eating it eventually.
- ❏ I will burn it off later.
- ❏ I will only have one piece.

- ❏ It is fat-free/low-calorie.
- ❏ I won't have this again for a long time.
- ❏ I do not usually eat this.
- ❏ I paid for it.
- ❏ Healthy food doesn't taste as good.
- ❏ I'm big-boned.
- ❏ It's genetic—I'm just born this way.
- ❏ It won't matter.
- ❏ I did not eat lunch (breakfast, dinner), so I am making up for it.
- ❏ Other _____ _____

This strategy allows your child to be aware of each checked-off excuse. When she experiences a rationalization, she can remind herself that there are alternative behaviors that she can consider. Over time, it is possible to make positive changes to rationalization habits. Understanding the many excuses she makes will allow your child to catch herself when these issues show up, to hold herself accountable, and to focus on how she really wants to be behaving.

BALANCED THINKING

Create Power Cards to Effectively Process Thoughts

Now that you know more about the self-sabotaging thoughts that plague us most often, we will further examine and challenge our thinking. Your child can use an extremely helpful tool, "power cards," to accomplish this. A power card is one way of identifying and documenting an unhelpful thought (e.g., "I am bored, so I am going to grab a snack") and then coming up with replies to help avoid giving in to it (e.g., "Just because I'm bored doesn't mean I need to overeat. I could find something better to do"). Power cards can be created using three-by-five-inch index cards or by jotting notes in a smartphone, computer, or tablet.

Some kids choose to make one for every unhelpful thought they experience; that way they will be fully equipped for any situation. This is ideal if your child is open to it. He can also start with the most pressing ones that he experiences most frequently and add on over time as he notices others. If using index cards, I recommend laminating the cards he carries with him so that he is better prepared when unhelpful thoughts surface.

If you notice your child is reluctant to write on the index cards—perhaps because he doesn't like writing, he doesn't want to put into writing thoughts that may evoke shame or guilt, or he is afraid he will lose or misplace the cards—try a few for yourself first. Then sit down with your child and ask him to give it a try. Doing it together may ease some of his worries. You can also discuss possible replies aloud or use your smartphone or computer to record the conversation as opposed to writing out the power cards.

Do whatever helps your kid or teen maintain his healthy practice. Be open to alternative and creative methods of structuring the strategy. As long as your child is engaged with you and the material, be open to what works best for him.

Strategy 1, Strategy 20, and Strategy 21 have helped you and your child pinpoint the common, unhelpful excuses that are derailing his health plans. Now is the moment to challenge that kind of thinking so he can make better choices. For example, before a special occasion such as a birthday party, where tempting foods such as pizza, birthday cake, or sodas are expected, he can anticipate thoughts and rationalizations he is likely to experience. Then, in the moment, he can draw on the helpful responses he brainstormed on his power card to increase his chances of success in engaging in healthful behaviors. If he is feeling particularly nervous, he can bring the power card along with him and duck into the bathroom to review it before the food is served.

EXERCISE: Making Power Cards

Show your child the following examples of power cards. Try writing a few yourself; then ask him to sit down with a pen or pencil and index cards and get started.

POWER CARD

UNHELPFUL THOUGHT:

I am bored, so I am going to eat.

HELPFUL REPLY:

1. I could choose to occupy myself and find something to do.

2. So what if I am bored? That does not mean I have to overeat.

3. I could feel bored and feel like I want to snack and still choose not to snack before bed.

4. I could choose to be bored and overeat, but that will lead me to feeling ashamed and lead me away from my health and fitness goals.

5. Am I really bored, or am I avoiding something and making food my distraction?

POWER CARD

UNHELPFUL THOUGHT:

This will never work for me.

HELPFUL REPLY:

1. I have never really made the commitment and followed a plan the way I needed to. It is possible that if I stick to it, this experience will be different because of all that I am putting into it.

2. In the past that thought led me to give up, not follow through with my plan and achieve my goals. This time I'm going to give it my all!

3. If I have a negative attitude, it is going to affect my mood. It is important that I stay positive and motivated.

4. I know that when I have put in effort to accomplish things, I am generally successful. There is no reason that I can't be successful at this.

5. I have as good a chance as anyone to succeed.

6. I will have some better moments and some more challenging ones. That is what life is all about. The challenging moments will pass.

POWER CARD

UNHELPFUL THOUGHT:

It's not fair that I have to work toward achieving my health and fitness goals.

HELPFUL REPLIES:

1. I could focus on how fair or unfair it is, but how is this going to lead me to success with my goals?

2. Life isn't fair. We each have our individual challenges. This is mine, and it may be something different for someone else.

3. Most people do have to work at achieving success in their health and fitness goals.

4. People who are more healthful eat and behave differently from those who eat and behave unhealthily (they eat smaller portions, eat only when they are hungry, are more active, etc.).

5. This negative thinking leads me to give in to my unhelpful thoughts and make excuses for my behavior. I need to be mindful of my choices and be open and self-aware. I have the power to make better choices.

POWER CARD

UNHELPFUL THOUGHT:
I will only have one piece of this food.

HELPFUL REPLY:

1. From my past experiences, I usually do not stop at just eating one piece. I usually end up eating a lot more than I intended.

2. These pieces are just more calories. All the calories add up.

3. One piece leads me to eat more because I want to feel satisfied and find that it does not happen until I'm full or overstuffed.

4. When I do not give in to these thoughts, it helps to empower me and allows me to believe that I can do it if I try. This positive thinking motivates me to achieve my goals.

5. One piece of something sweet, salty, or crunchy compels me to have many other pieces of sweet, salty, or crunchy foods. I usually don't stop at one portion.

By making power cards, your child can establish what rationalizations tend to come up, reframe the way he thinks about them, and impose more mindful, balanced thinking, which will ultimately impact his behavior.

🧳 CHECK YOUR BAGGAGE

We all sometimes put ourselves down for the way we think, especially when we make decisions we regret. We even get upset for getting down on ourselves! We're our own worst critics. It never surprises me that when I ask my clients what they consider their negative attributes, they answer quickly and emphatically. When I ask about positive qualities, they take a lot longer to answer and often have a much shorter list. We readily point out the negative parts of ourselves because, unfortunately, those stand out for us.

Though you've certainly taught your children many things over the years, you may have overlooked teaching them how to handle their negative thoughts, especially if you sometimes struggle with some of the same issues they do and have never learned how to do it yourself. Knowing that may evoke feelings of disappointment or regret because you didn't make those connections for them or because you relate so personally.

When you picked up this book, you were not expected to know how to handle negative thoughts if you were never taught before. How wonderful that you're giving yourself and your child that gift! You are facilitating critical skills that will benefit you and your child for a lifetime. The added benefit is that these skills can easily apply to other areas of challenge, as well.

With time and practice, you and your child will come to recognize thoughts as simply thoughts, instead of as absolute truths. Ultimately, if you tell yourself you can't change, that life's not fair, and that you're bored and need to overeat, you'll buy in to those sentiments—and your child probably will, too. Alongside your child, recognize that your thoughts are only thoughts; gently, compassionately accept that the thoughts are there. Process them. Study them with interest and inquisitiveness. Then you'll both be able to make more meaningful decisions.

This journey explores the many facets of who we are. Part of lifelong health and wellness is to learn to appreciate ourselves at the core and to make changes that meet our needs. Through this process, you and your child will learn that *thoughts and feelings are something you have, rather than something you are.*

REVIEW

Your thinking about eating and exercise will always prompt certain behaviors. Sometimes these are not in line with the way you truly want to act or based on your values and goals. It is important to evaluate if that is the case, so that you can work to make well-thought-out, mindful decisions.

Kids and teens should continually evaluate:

- Thoughts
- Triggers
- Rationalizations
- How they behave based on thoughts and feelings
- How they will think and feel if they behave that way
- How they might think and feel if they behave differently
- The stinking thinking that may be getting in the way of healthy eating and exercising
- The rationalizations used to justify behavior
- How they are feeling in general (physically, emotionally, and socially) and how that may be affecting their decision making.

Kids and teens should continue to:

- Recognize that thoughts and feelings are not facts
- Create as many power cards as are helpful to support the process
- Feel hopeful and celebrate that they have a choice!

 MINDFULNESS EXERCISE: Accepting Yourself

See page 221 for the mindfulness exercise that corresponds to this chapter, and refer to page 217 for instructions on accessing the audio.

5

The Power of the 4Ps

This is just too hard. I tried to lose weight in the past, and I just can't keep it going. I keep tripping up, especially when I'm out with friends or at a family occasion or holiday. —CRAIG, AGE 19

I tend to be hungry most of the time. I usually settle on grabbing a bite at the cafeteria at school—it's just more convenient. What they offer are the typical fast foods. I recognize it's not the best choice, but it's easy, and I'm hungry. —PAIGE, AGE 18

THE 4PS ARE FOUR STEPS—predicting, planning, putting the plan into action, and practicing—that will help families achieve both short- and long-term goals for health and wellness. By expecting challenges (because they'll always show up) and working through them with the 4Ps, we can all live healthier, more satisfied, and more meaningful lives. A key facet of the 4Ps is to *practice, practice, practice,* because change takes time. As always, it's also important for parents to practice what you preach here.

1. **PREDICTING**

   We go through our lives anticipating what's going to come next. It is so natural and normal that you likely never even think about it. For kids and teens who struggle with eating and exercise, anticipation is even more important. Adults know that thoughts and feelings ebb and flow and are not always consistent and predictable, but it can and should become second nature for kids and teens to think ahead about challenges that might come up during the day and how they might react. These are not thoughts that come about in a hyper-focused, obsessive way, but rather in a mindful and thoughtful way.

The comprehensive process of self-evaluation discussed in Chapters 3 and 4 provided insight as to what challenges might present themselves. Within this framework, parents and kids and teens can work together to predict what might trip them up. Having this self-awareness is the first step toward making a plan, committing to take direct action, and practicing healthier skills day in and day out.

2. PLANNING

Plan by creating strategies that reinforce core values on a daily basis, and be prepared when challenges arise (these skills were established in Chapter 2).

Once your child has a pretty good idea of what challenges may appear, together you can come up with a plan that supports your child's daily practice and long-term goals. Your child can decide on strategies that seem realistic and most promising and stick with them throughout the day when faced with challenges.

3. PUTTING THE PLAN INTO ACTION

Your child puts the plan into action consistently when challenges arise. Even though your child's first impulse may be to do what they have always done in various situations, your child can stick with the plan and take note of how they think and feel while following through with it. Nothing is set in stone, and transition, adjustment, and evolution are expected and inevitable, so the plan may very well need to be recalibrated from time to time. Remember, making this a practice is key and requires a consistent effort and openness to the process. Along the way, there will be some more challenging and effortful days and others that are more seamless; your child is to forge ahead no matter how easy or difficult it seems. The steps to effective problem solving are explained herein.

4. PRACTICING

Your child will practice the skills and commit to a healthful life. Among the topics in this chapter are behavioral change and proactive engagement. These are the essence of what allows kids and teens to empower themselves: proactively problem solving, not only when they are faced with challenging situations, but also on a daily basis.

In this chapter, you'll find relatable examples of circumstances that may prove tricky and guidance on how to implement specific behavior changes. Examples include working through cravings, eating healthfully and mindfully, and avoiding succumbing to peer pressure.

Even after predicting, planning, putting into action, and practicing, challenges may arise for which your child or teen did not adequately plan. For those circumstances, using effective problem-solving skills to work through barriers to healthful eating and behavior can be helpful. As a bonus, these same skills apply to many of life's future challenges.

STRATEGY 23

PREDICT

Encourage Self-Acceptance

Your child's commitment to getting to know himself well and being accepting of himself is key. As pointed out in Chapter 1, our propensity is to avoid uncomfortable thoughts and feelings and be disapproving of the parts of ourselves that we do not like. We resist being accepting of ourselves.

Many people believe that in order to be accepting of ourselves, we need to fully and positively embrace *all* aspects of ourselves at all times. But self-acceptance rarely, if ever, starts out that way. It is typically built over time, as people gain confidence and mastery in the abilities that are meaningful to them. Their focus then shifts from a place of longing, sadness, or anger to a place of acknowledging, personal satisfaction, and gratitude. *You and your child, like all humans, are deserving of love, being valued, and being treated with respect.* It's a mantra that may be a new way of looking at yourself and the people you interact with.

I have observed, in my practice with clients and in the focus groups I ran when conducting research for this book, that teens need self-compassion, self-love, and self-confidence to be accepting of themselves. In one focus group, when the topic of fat shaming and bullying came up, most of the overweight teens reported having endured prolonged bullying at school; they all had their own painful stories. But it was evident that when something "clicked" for those teens, they were finally able to build up enough confidence and put resources in place to assert themselves, and the bullying stopped.

This particular focus group was attended by teens who had weight and health challenges as well as several others who did not. One of the teen boys from the latter category suddenly became exasperated and said, "What's wrong with you guys? Why didn't you stick up for yourselves? You see what happened when you did; [the teasing] stopped. I don't get you. I would never let that happen to me."

Another teen chimed in and reminded the boy that he was well built and muscular, which contributed to why he wasn't picked on. The other kids patiently sat and poignantly explained to him and a few others what had compelled them to stay quiet, feel hopeless, and buy into the belief that they weren't good enough. They were also able to explain what they actively did to build their confidence and take action toward self-acceptance and self-compassion/self-love.

What is self-acceptance? My definition is: *Self-acceptance is fully assessing and acknowledging yourself, challenging and changing the aspects of yourself that you have the power to, and accepting those aspects of yourself that you can't—while openly being with your challenges, your thoughts, and your feelings, whether or not they evoke discomfort. It is also recognizing that these challenges, thoughts, and feelings are part of you but not all of you and don't define who you are as a person. You get to decide who you are.*

As your child goes through this book's process of self-exploration and self-acceptance, he will more readily predict what daily practices he will need to pay attention to and put in place. He will learn about himself in relation to his thoughts and feelings (discussed in Chapters 1 and 5), his prior experiences and behaviors (discussed in Chapter 3), and his biological, psychological, and social makeup (discussed in Chapter 8). With maturity, he will become more flexible and open to learning, changing, growing, and maintaining his health.

EXERCISE: Review Your Challenges

To help your child recognize his challenges and predict and plan accordingly, have him fill out the following chart.

AREAS OF CHALLENGE	HOW THEY SHOW UP FOR ME
Negative thoughts about myself (e.g., I don't finish what I start, I'm lazy, etc.)	
Eating behavior (e.g., I overeat, hide food, etc.)	
Exercise behavior (e.g., I don't want to try anything new, I don't consistently exercise, etc.)	
Hunger (e.g., I get really hungry late at night, I skip meals and am left famished, etc.)	
Triggers (e.g., I'm triggered by smells of food, how I'm feeling physically, etc.)	
Cravings (e.g., I crave chocolate and peanut butter, etc.)	
Emotional eating (e.g., I overeat when I'm lonely and bored, etc.)	
Stinking thinking (e.g., I tend to have all-or-nothing or catastrophizing thinking, etc.)	
Rationalization (e.g., I tend to think that I'll only have one piece of cake or that I need it, etc.)	
Circumstances (e.g., peer pressure, family stress, physical condition, etc.)	

Everyone's challenges present differently, and at any point in time they can change or evolve. With acceptance comes an understanding that a challenge will not diminish unless effort is put in to make specific behavioral changes.

For example, you know that your child tends to crave ice cream after a soccer game because the team congregates at the local ice-cream store after the weekend games. You also know that your child tends to get two scoops of chocolate chunk ice cream with mounds of toppings on a sugar cone—even though he is aware there are more healthful alternatives at the shop. When the upcoming spring season arrives, your child rationalizes that it will be different this time and he won't get tempted to get the ice cream he typically rewards himself with for playing a good game.

Remind your child to predict his behavior based on what he knows about his challenges. Help him accept that if he doesn't plan ahead, he will most likely fall into the same behavior pattern and will opt for a familiar choice. If he learns to predict his behavior, he can effectively plan for an alternative or find a way to eat what he wants to, but more mindfully. He may opt for one scoop of ice cream instead of two, frozen yogurt or sorbet instead of ice cream, fewer toppings or an alternative such as fruit, or a cup instead of the sugar cone. He could also choose to vary his selection each time he goes there. Planning ahead gives him the opportunity to recognize that there are viable alternatives and that he has the power to make healthful choices.

PLAN

Create a Blueprint

Planning anything takes time and effort. It involves thinking ahead, coming up with a strategy, and being proactive in finding ways to effectively execute the plan. As the saying goes, *People don't plan to fail; they fail to plan.* Your child can take concrete steps to effectively plan to deal with a health-sabotaging situation before it arrives. Challenges are inevitable; therefore, it is critical and prudent to plan for them. Guide your child by informing her of these factors to consider when planning:

- **P**ay attention to your feelings and thought patterns
- **L**isten to what your body is telling you
- **A**ssess your potential challenges
- **N**otice your intuition
- **N**ote your worst-case scenario
- **I**magine your best-case scenario
- **N**urture balanced thinking
- **G**enerate a concrete plan

PAY ATTENTION TO YOUR FEELINGS AND THOUGHT PATTERNS

At times, our thoughts and feelings can definitely be irrational and unpredictable (discussed in detail in Chapter 1). Helping your child pay attention to her feelings and thought patterns while she is planning will inform you how challenging a situation may be for her and will help her plan to succeed. For example, if your child is feeling down because she got a poor grade in a subject she really cares about, that may detract from her planning and being mindfully focused when she attends a party the same evening. By being aware of her emotional state, she'll be better prepared at the party.

LISTEN TO WHAT YOUR BODY IS TELLING YOU

Your child also needs to "listen" for what's showing up in her body. Because our physiology directly affects the rest of our body, if your child is experiencing aches, sensations, or some other physiological reaction, this, too, may affect her healthful efforts.

ASSESS YOUR POTENTIAL CHALLENGES

Your child should evaluate the challenges that keep her from carrying out her healthful behaviors. These may include potential cravings, hunger, etc. When formulating a plan, consider these factors to increase the likelihood that the plan will be created, that it will be helpful, and that it will be carried out.

NOTICE YOUR INTUITION

Your child's intuition is also noteworthy. It is her hunch or gut feeling that may clue her in to emotional factors she might not have otherwise considered. For example, your child expresses feeling an unusual sense of dread about going to a family dinner and is worried about planning for it. She can't quite put her finger on what's coming up but knows there's something there. Through deeper exploration, she discovers that she's angry at her uncle for something her uncle said to her during the last family dinner, which she feels bad about because she never addressed it.

NOTE YOUR WORST-CASE SCENARIO

When your child anticipates the worst-case scenario in a situation, she is able to evaluate potential risks and gauge how best to behave in line with her values. For example, if she's attending a party to watch a major sporting event, she's fully aware that there will be many less-nutritious food choices available, and she will experience multiple triggers that will make it extremely challenging for her to eat mindfully. If she anticipates the worst-case scenario, which would include *all* of her craving foods being right there at her disposal, she can effectively plan for how she will handle that situation.

IMAGINE YOUR BEST-CASE SCENARIO

On the other hand, if she imagines the best-case scenario, she can contemplate the possible rewards of the situation. In the case of the party, she can list the more nutritious food choices she will mindfully choose to eat and consider how satisfied she will feel, both physically and emotionally, after doing so.

NURTURE BALANCED THINKING

Balanced thinking means considering a plan from both an intellectual and an emotional point of view. For example, when your child attends a big Fourth of July barbecue, she's able to plan for her mind telling her, "Eat everything in sight because you never know when you'll be at a barbecue again," and reframe it as, "You have a grill at home. If you ever want something grilled, it's easy enough to do."

EXERCISE: Generate a Concrete Plan

Planning should be centered on your child's values and specific goals and objectives. As will be discussed further in Chapter 6, long-term goals should be SMART (**S**pecific, **M**easurable, **A**ction-Oriented, **R**ealistic, and **T**ime-Based).

After explaining the planning process to your child, ask her to assess how she would plan for a given situation. Have her look at all the different elements.

SITUATION YOU ARE PLANNING FOR:

_____

_____

_____

_____

HOW MIGHT THESE ELEMENTS IMPACT YOUR PLANNING?

Feelings and thought patterns: _____

_____

Body: _____

_____

Potential challenges: _____

_____

_____

Intuition: _____

_____

Imagining a worst-case scenario: _____

_____

Imagining a best-case scenario: _____

_____

Balanced thinking: _____

_____

The actual plan: _____

_____

Next, you and your child will explore effective problem-solving methods to put into action behaviors that are in line with her values and goals. Becoming a master problem solver affords her the skills to successfully handle any situation that may come her way.

PUT YOUR PLAN INTO ACTION

Become a Master Problem Solver in Six Steps

Skills build upon each other. Once your child is able to predict and plan for situations as they arise, he can get ready to problem solve and take direct action in each situation. Taking action isn't just about doing something—here you'll help your child **A**scertain the challenge; **C**ommit to being specific and accurate about the situation; **T**hink about possible solutions; **I**nvestigate the potential fallout of each solution; **O**bjectively choose a solution; and **N**ow, put your solution into action. For example, even though your child is generally eating nutritiously and mindfully at home, he's asked you for help because lunch at school has become challenging.

Together you predict, based on his prior behavior, that he will opt for less-healthful choices when they are available; he will eat whatever his friends are eating because he doesn't want to stand out as being different; he will eat more than he intended because of his typical rationalization, "It tastes so good, I might as well eat as much as I want to." You can help him plan for and put into action a strategy for eating lunch at school.

THE CHALLENGE: EATING AT SCHOOL

- **A**scertain the challenge as quickly as possible: *eating healthfully at the high school cafeteria.*
- **C**ommit to being specific and accurate. *Food options are limited and mostly high-fat; less-nutritious foods are offered.*
- **T**hink through the array of possible solutions. *Bring your own food to school; eat smaller portions of the food items at school; advocate for healthier choices at school.*
- **I**nvestigate the implications of each solution. *You or your parent would need to prepare lunch every day; even though you're eating*

*smaller portions of the foods at school, they are still not the most
healthful choices, and you may be left feeling hungry; your peers or
school's administration may resist your initiatives to make changes.*

- **O**bjectively choose the best solution(s). *Plan to bring your own
fruit and vegetables to school, have a small portion of the protein
the school is offering for the day, and in the future plan to advocate
for the school to provide a variety of healthful alternatives, such as
low-fat yogurt, whole wheat and multigrain bread for sandwiches,
and low-fat milk to drink.*

- **N**ow, act on the solution. *Bring in a banana and carrot sticks
from home and eat the grilled chicken your school offers; speak
to school administrators and form a committee to bring healthier
options to school and keep healthy lunch foods/fruit available.*

In another example, let's say you're all going to a cousin's wedding.
Your child predicts, based on his prior experiences, that buffets are
challenging because he tends to overeat and finds himself eating impulsively. He also recognizes that cream-filled wedding cake is typically
served for dessert. Even though he normally feels full after the meal, he
usually indulges in more than one portion of dessert and rationalizes
that it's a special occasion; he should eat wedding cake to celebrate
with his cousin and should eat as much as he feels like. Together you
help him plan for and put into action a strategy for eating mindfully at
the wedding.

THE CHALLENGE: GOING TO A COUSIN'S WEDDING

- **A**scertain the challenge as quickly as possible: *eating from a
buffet at your cousin's wedding.*
- **C**ommit to being specific and accurate. *Food options are
plentiful, and you tend to eat quickly and impulsively, which leads
to overeating.*
- **T**hink through the array of possible solutions. *Eat before the
wedding; mindfully eat at the wedding, and pay attention to eating
slowly; read your hunger and fullness cues.*
- **I**nvestigate the implications of each solution. *You would need
to make time to prepare and eat beforehand; you may feel paying
attention so intently may take away from being in the moment at
the wedding.*

- **O**bjectively choose the best solution(s). *Eat a small snack before the wedding so you don't come to the wedding starving; mindfully eat at the wedding while paying attention to eating slowly and pacing yourself between foods and courses.*
- **N**ow act on the solution. *Eat a baked sweet potato and some pita chips with hummus before the wedding, skip the appetizers because you're still digesting the food from home and feel satiated, and have a small to moderate portion of the main course and a small, satisfying sliver of wedding cake.*

EXERCISE: Take ACTION

Ask your child to select a food situation that can be challenging. Use these six steps to take ACTION and problem solve through the challenge.

- **A**scertain the challenge as quickly as possible. The challenge is:

  _____

- **C**ommit to being specific and accurate _____

  _____

- **T**hink through the array of possible solutions _____

  _____

- **I**nvestigate the implications of each solution _____

  _____

- **O**bjectively choose the best solution or variations of solutions

  _____

- **N**ow, act on the solution _____

  _____

Your child will use problem-solving skills to work through barriers to healthful eating and behavior. He should evaluate the effectiveness of his approach and make changes to it as necessary. As a parent you may want to explore and be open to other integrative problem-solving methods that may effectively work for your child.[54] As with anything else, to effectively accomplish a goal and do something well, he'll need to put time and effort into an approach and continually practice. If this practice is consistent, it will guide his behavior all day, every day.

PRACTICE, PRACTICE, PRACTICE

Reinforce Your Skills

Most people look for a quick weight-loss fix through some magical diet or gimmick. A market data report stated that in 2013, the US weight-loss market was a staggering $60.5 billion industry. Included in this number were diet soft drinks, artificial sweeteners, health clubs, commercial weight-loss chains, meal replacements (shakes) and diet pills, diet websites and apps, medical programs (weight-loss surgery, doctors, hospitals/clinic programs, prescription diet drugs, bariatrician plans, very low-calorie diet programs (where all meals are replaced), low-calorie dinner entrees, diet books, and exercise DVDs.[55] The weight loss from extreme diets is often temporary, with weight gain to inevitably follow. By some estimates, as many as 80 percent of overweight people who manage to slim down noticeably after a diet gain some or all of the weight back within one year.[56]

In a 2007 study, Traci Mann at the University of Minnesota and her coauthors conducted a comprehensive and rigorous analysis of diet studies, analyzing thirty-one long-term studies. When asked what happens to people on diets in the long run, she responded, "Would they have been better off to not go on a diet at all? We decided to dig up and analyze every study that followed people on diets for two to five years. We concluded most of them would have been better off not going on the diet at all. Their weight would be pretty much the same, and their bodies would not suffer the wear and tear from losing weight and gaining it all back."[57]

These studies show that between one-third to two-thirds of dieters regain more weight than they lost on their diets. It is even likely that the extent to which dieting is counterproductive is underestimated in these studies. A. Janet Tomiyama, a coauthor of the study, commented that several findings indicate that dieting is actually a consistent predictor of future weight gain. She also said that one study found that both men and women who participated in formal weight-loss programs gained significantly more weight over a two-year period than those who had not participated in a weight-loss program.

In a 2015 study of 800 healthy adults, researchers from the Weizmann Institute of Science found that, biologically, people respond differently to eating the same meal. Tailoring meal plans to individuals' biology may be

107

the future of dieting. Dieting hasn't been effective because it doesn't take individuals' unique physiology into account.[58]

When looking at teens and young adults, the weight-amplifying effect of dieting was evaluated in a novel study on more than 2,000 sets of twins from Finland, ages sixteen to twenty-five.[59] The results of the study indicated that dieting itself, independent of genetics, is significantly associated with accelerated weight gain *and* increased the risk of becoming overweight. The researchers concluded, "It is now well established that the more people engage in dieting, the more they gain weight in the long term."

Other research on nearly 17,000 kids, ages nine to fourteen, also found that dieting was a significant predictor of weight gain.[60] Moreover, the risk of binge eating increased with the frequency of dieting. Boys and girls who dieted frequently were five and twelve times, respectively, more likely to report binge eating compared to their non-dieting counterparts. The researchers concluded that "in the long term, dieting to control weight is not only ineffective, it may actually promote weight gain." In yet another study, teenage dieters had twice the risk of becoming overweight compared to non-dieting teens.[61] Dieting also appears to be causally linked to both obesity and eating disorders in adolescents and teens.[62]

You may find your child caught up in the vicious cycle of dieting, which is an ineffective and counterproductive means to maintain healthful eating and exercise behaviors in the long run. She may get stuck in the same rut that so many others find themselves in. After starting her first diet, she was probably successful at losing some weight. Biologically, however, her body experienced the dieting as a form of deprivation and starvation. Her cells didn't know she was voluntarily restricting her food intake. Her body shifted into survival mode, her metabolism slowed down, and her food cravings escalated. With each diet, her body learned and adapted, resulting in rebound weight gain. Consequently, she's left feeling that she failed and is, therefore, a failure. This is a deflating cycle, leaving her feeling frustrated, disappointed, and hopeless.

The secret to lifelong healthful behaviors is found in our daily decision making and consistent practice. It is not about diets and quick fixes. Research has substantiated that diets just don't work and are not appropriate for kids and teens. We can't will ourselves into being a star athlete or being a top professional without sustainable practice. *"Will may be the power, but it's nothing without the practice."*[63]

Just as professional baseball players (or any athletes) continually spend many hours practicing even though they are skilled and seasoned, so do we need to practice if we want to continually sharpen and maintain our skills and effectively continue healthful behaviors. Just as we continually take care of a car and commit to its routine maintenance, such as bringing it in for an oil change so that it runs properly, the same goes for our bodies. We also need to take direct action and provide constant care and maintenance to ensure that our organs, muscles, and joints function well and will not break down when we need them.

EXERCISE: Practicing Your Skills: Going to a Party

Time has to be made to practice skills daily. As with anything, the more your child practices a task, the more easily she'll perform it and the better she'll become at it. Your child will evaluate the actions from Strategy 25, prepare, try them out, and adjust by considering the example of going to a party.

- Identify, predict, and plan for emotional stressors that may negatively impact your eating behavior (your mood, fears or concerns, etc.).
- Because of the likelihood of overeating, before going to the party, take a look at the restaurant menu or ask the hostess what they're serving. You will have the benefit of being informed and can make the choice to either eat prior, eat what is at the party because there are healthy options, or make some other choice.
- Try to identify things that you can do (other than eating) when you are feeling a strong urge to overeat (e.g., speak with a friend, go for a walk, or drink a cold or hot beverage).
- Practice by periodically reading your power cards (see Chapter 4), engaging in encouraging self-talk, practicing your mindfulness skills, acknowledging and taking a daily inventory of ways you demonstrated your core value of health, putting a support person in place so that you can reach out to them when you need some reassurance or guidance, etc.

List additional things you may proactively do to practice your skills.

_____

_____

_____

It is not enough just to learn about the 4Ps. Your child has to *do* them. It entails a lifelong commitment so that healthful behavior becomes habit, just like brushing one's teeth on a daily basis.

Many people think it takes just twenty-one days to change or develop a new habit, but one recent study suggests that the average might be closer to sixty-six days or even longer—especially if a habit is particularly hard to pick up or if the person trying to make a change is habit resistant.[64] However long it takes, it's important to remember that learning anything new—from playing the piano to making a presentation at school—requires repetition and persistence, two things you and your child will need to constantly reinforce on this journey.

CHECK YOUR BAGGAGE

In this chapter you and your child were introduced to the 4Ps—predict, plan, put into action, and practice. With the 4Ps, you can create a blueprint for dealing with challenging situations as they arise. You can predict what may be a barrier to healthful behavior, adequately plan for it, act upon the plan, and practice the cumulative skills in this book every day until they become routine and a way of life. Observe your own behavior and assess if you are "practicing what you preach." Are you carrying out the healthy behaviors that you are asking your child to commit to? You might be confronted with your own challenges and areas of "stuckness."

Self-acceptance is accepting *all* of ourselves, which can sometimes prove challenging. We all contain disorganized parts of ourselves. Self-reflection around these may evoke feelings of shame, disappointment, and regret, which are all natural. By working to improve your own self-image, you can better model those skills for your child.

Recognize that you can be instrumental in helping your child effectively plan and problem solve through challenges. Your own behavior can set your child up with a template. If a given solution is not readily apparent, exercise patience and help lead and guide your child to various options so that he or she can learn to see the full scope of alternatives.

Throughout this process, you can choose to share challenging situations that arise for you, as well. Giving examples from your own life may normalize things for your child, so that she or he may be more likely to open up to you. It may not always come easily for you as a parent to be vulnerable and express your private and personal thoughts and feelings. Take it one step at a time, and be aware of how you may be reacting to sharing. Your body language, tone of voice, the content of what you are expressing, and many other factors may directly impact your child's willingness to share. If this is challenging or uncomfortable for you, you may want to share that feeling with your child, too, so that your child internalizes that it is okay to be imperfect and experience discomfort.

Living healthfully is a process. Recognize that sometimes, although you intend to keep the momentum going, you may slip up. This is common. There is always room to work on these techniques and integrate what is meaningful to you on an ongoing basis. If you are feeling a greater sense of empowerment and self-love, it will serve you well and help you join your child in making a lifelong change.

 REVIEW

You learned how to cope with challenging situations as they arise by implementing the 4Ps. You explored how to work toward self-acceptance, plan for and consider certain factors as they come up, and problem solve and put into action the solution that works best in a given situation. There is no quick fix or shortcut to achieving healthful behaviors. Healthy living entails putting in conscious time and effort.

Kids and teens can:

- Predict what thoughts, feelings, bodily sensations, and behaviors may be challenging.
- Create a blueprint for change.
- Use the six steps to problem solving to work through given challenges: ascertaining the challenge, committing to being specific and accurate, thinking through the array of possible solutions, investigating the implications of each solution, objectively choosing the best solution, and acting on the solution.
- Make daily decisions to practice healthy behaviors, promoting lifelong and consistent change.

 MINDFULNESS EXERCISE: Striving for What You Want

See page 222 for the mindfulness exercise that corresponds to this chapter, and refer to page 217 for instructions on accessing the audio.

6

All in the Family:
What Parents Can Do

My parents just don't understand me. They're always telling me what I can and can't eat. It's embarrassing. They also compare me with other kids. Now, that's really supposed to make me feel good. Like my dad is one to talk—we sit down at a restaurant, and he goes straight for the bread. He can't help himself. I wonder where I get it from.

—JARED, AGE 15

I find myself feeling protective of my daughter Olivia but also really angry at her that she can't control herself. Most of my friends' kids are able to wear anything they want, but we have to be selective when we go shopping. It brings me to tears when I see how much she suffers. Her self-esteem is being affected, and she sometimes stays at home instead of going out with friends. I'm worried about her, feel responsible for this, and feel angry with her all at the same time.

—LIZ, PARENT

No MAN IS AN ISLAND, so even though kids and teens want to be independent, it's impossible to talk about their lives and habits without also examining those of their families. Family exerts a powerful influence over the ways in which we think, feel, and behave in regard to our eating and exercise. This chapter discusses some of the ways in which parents may consciously or subconsciously influence their children. It also tackles some of the most common and complicated scenarios (e.g., hiding food) at the intersection of parenting and wellness.

We'll look at how family sets the stage for healthful habits, including the ways in which messages are transmitted regarding food, health, and weight, how these messages affect children, and how to be more

cognizant of these critical messages so that you are conveying encouragement, care, and parental support.

Even when all is going well, it takes time to develop new habits and
ways of thinking, so an important part of this chapter will be learning to
assess whether your family is working collaboratively as a team. You will
also learn to give the kind of support your child needs in order to increase
the probability of success on your child's healthful journey.

I ask you as parents to participate in a self-evaluation in order to
understand your own relationship with food and how that affects how
you are raising your own children. You'll determine how and if you are
modeling healthy eating and exercising behaviors to your children and
what messages you're conveying.

No matter where kids and teens are in this journey, it's never too late to
get started making changes. It takes an effort to prepare healthier, more
nutritious meals, and getting into the practice of exercising regularly isn't
something that happens overnight. These changes take time but are well
worth it for the sake of your entire family's health and well-being.

STRATEGY 27

MIRROR, MIRROR ON THE WALL

Model Healthful Behaviors

The best thing to do to get your child to practice healthful behaviors is to
model what you're expecting from her. Kids dislike hypocrisy. They do not
like to be judged and criticized—or watch you do that to other people. It
can make them concerned that you may be harboring those thoughts and
feelings about them. This in turn makes them less likely to share with you
and trust that they can turn to you when they need help.

If you are overweight or obese yourself, it increases the likelihood that
your child will be, as well. Parental weight is a significant predictor of a
child's weight, particularly among seven- to fifteen-year-olds.[65] The commitment to helping your child is also a positive way to help yourself and
benefit your whole family.

A way to assess whether you are modeling the behavior you expect
from your child is by taking time for some introspection. Make sure that
what you are advocating and asking for is in line with what you are actually doing, not just saying. A general question to ask yourself is, "What
have I been teaching my child by my actions?" This includes actions you

113

take toward eating, fitness, and health in general, as well as how you communicate with your partner and others.

The intent here is not to place blame on you, the parent, as the impetus for why your child is facing challenges or behaving the way that she is. Rather, it's to empower you to recognize that you are an important, if not the most important, person in your child's life and can make a substantial difference in helping to facilitate change. Your family dynamics are just one piece of the puzzle contributing to your child's health.

———

EXERCISE: Assess Yourself as a Role Model

This exercise is for parents. Ask yourself the following questions to assess whether you are modeling the behaviors you expect from your child and to learn to be more mindful in your thoughts and behaviors:

YOUR ACTIONS

- Are you exercising regularly?
- Are you eating healthfully?
- Are you doing things that send messages to your child regarding your body image (such as weighing yourself incessantly, getting frustrated because your clothing is tight, etc.)?

YOUR COMMUNICATION

- What are you communicating about yourself? (e.g., "I'm so fat, I can't stand it" or "This bathing suit makes me look so enormous."). Your child is hearing you make self-deprecating judgments about yourself in regard to your weight and body size.
- What are you communicating about your partner? (e.g., "Haven't you had enough?" or "That will go straight to your thighs."). Your child is hearing you make judgments of others in regard to their eating behaviors and body size.
- What are you communicating about people in general? (e.g., "That woman must have no self-control" or "Doesn't she care that she looks like that?"). Your child is hearing you make judgments of others in regard to their level of motivation and appearance.

- Are you complimenting or commenting on other people's weight? (e.g., "You look great —how much weight did you lose?" or "She would be so pretty if she lost some weight."). Your child is hearing you make judgments about the value of others based on their body size and appearance.

WAYS TO BE MORE MINDFUL

Pay attention to:
- Your biases and judgments toward yourself and others;
- The level of frustration and anger you feel when you're thinking about your own health and fitness challenges and issues, or when you are confronted with others';
- What "stuckness" you have in regard to your own healthful behavior;
- How much space there is between what you think and how you decide to act.

Instead of impulsively behaving or saying what is on your mind, consider:
- Whether it is in line with your integrity,
- What consequences it will have for you and others,
- Alternative ways of acting or communicating.

It is essential that you are mindful not to criticize your body or the bodies of others in front of your child. You are the most important person in your child's life. If she sees that you disdain your body, it makes it easier for her to dislike hers. In the book *Like Mother, Like Daughter*, Deborah Waterhouse writes about the influence mothers have on their daughters' body image, but sons can be greatly affected by their parents' body-image issues, as well. You can challenge yourself and work proactively with your child to create a positive body image and increased self-love and self-compassion. This is a positive way to bond and foster mutual love and understanding.

115

YOU CAN DO IT

Examine Your Core Beliefs

Core beliefs are defined as fundamental, inflexible, absolute, and generalized beliefs that people hold about themselves, others, the world, and/or the future.[66] When a core belief is riddled with negativity, such as "I'm useless," it can have a profound effect on a child's self-concept and sense of self-efficacy. Self-efficacy is the strength of a child's belief that he has the ability to complete tasks and reach goals.[67] Based on social learning theory, what we know about self-efficacy is that it can be developed through mastery, social modeling, social persuasion, and mood. Individuals with strong self-efficacy view challenging problems as tasks to be mastered, have a greater interest in the activities they do, and recover quickly from setbacks.[68] In this way, self-efficacy can directly affect your child's willingness to integrate healthy changes and the extent to which he will practice the changes.

If your child has high self-efficacy, he's more likely to take on a challenge and stick to a plan, even in moments of frustration or adversity. By determining his beliefs regarding his power to affect situations, you and your child can understand how and why self-efficacy strongly influences his ability to face challenges and make positive choices along the way.

Core beliefs typically center on themes of lovability (e.g., "I am undesirable"), adequacy ("I am incompetent"), and/or helplessness (e.g., "I am trapped").[69] With a negative self-concept or core belief (the way we see ourselves), your child may believe that his situation can't change. This may lessen the chances that he will take action to make changes and stick with them over time.

Greater self-efficacy can be developed by building a child's confidence. Once you understand the family dynamics that perpetuate negative core beliefs, you can identify the skills and experiences needed to feel capable and effective at overcoming challenges.

Here are some examples of how core beliefs get influenced by family dynamics.

Nora is raised in a household with her parents and older sister, Karen. Karen is a cheerleader, very social, and a good student. She is also fortunate to have a fast metabolism and eats whatever she wants and remains thin. Nora is also a good student, but she isn't interested in sports and has been overweight throughout her childhood and adolescence. Nora and Karen have been treated significantly differently by their mother in regard to their eating behaviors. Nora is never allowed seconds on dessert at dinner, but Karen is; Nora's snacks are restricted, whereas Karen's are not; and Nora is constantly reminded that she should or shouldn't eat this or that, whereas Karen is encouraged to finish everything on her plate.

NORA'S CORE BELIEF: I am unlovable because I am overweight.

NORA'S THOUGHTS: If I were thin and able to have more control over my eating, then maybe I would be accepted by my mother, sister, and friends.

NORA'S FEELINGS: Sad, frustrated, and disappointed.

NORA'S BEHAVIOR: Nora hides food and snacks in her room because she feels deprived of them and eats them voraciously and impulsively to avoid her mother finding out.

TO HELP FACILITATE HIGHER SELF-EFFICACY: Nora's parents would foster a healthier household by having healthy foods readily accessible and holding the same standards for everyone. All members would be treated equally, with each having one mindfully portioned dessert. Additionally, they would be encouraged to eat only when they are physically hungry. Nora would learn to assess her hunger cues and would take personal responsibility for gauging that to build mastery, independence, and confidence in making healthful decisions.

Jake is growing up in a house with his parents, an older brother, and a younger sister. There are few boundaries set at home regarding food, discipline, and academics. Snacks are readily available and plentiful, and there are few restrictions as to when to eat them and the quantities to consume. Both parents are overweight, with his mother being obese. He and his siblings were taught to finish their plates and never waste food because it showed a lack of appreciation for being so fortunate to have it. Family outings are typically to restaurants, as opposed to an activity that centers on play or movement.

All children in the family are overweight, with Jake being the heaviest. He was never encouraged to try out for sports teams and

117

never attempted to, because he assumed he would never be good at them and would disappoint his teammates. Jake is chronically teased at school, especially by one "popular" child who continually refers to him as "Jake the whale." Nothing was ever done about it, because it always happens when teachers aren't around, and Jake is too embarrassed to tell anyone.

JAKE'S CORE BELIEF: I am ineffective. I can't do much of anything right. Even if I try, it will be useless. I'll never be able to change my circumstances.

JAKE'S THOUGHTS: No one wants me on their team. I'll mess it up for them, and who can blame them? If I were thinner and more attractive and less like my family members, then maybe I would be better at sports.

JAKE'S FEELINGS: Sad, frustrated, angry, and hopeless.

JAKE'S BEHAVIOR: Jake doesn't put a concerted effort into most of what he does. His grades are just marginally passing, he is sloppy and disorganized, and he continues to be challenged with portion-control issues and eating less healthful foods.

TO HELP FACILITATE HIGHER SELF-EFFICACY: Jake's family would meet with a nutritionist or attend nutrition workshops to learn about general healthful eating and how to maintain a healthy household. They would portion out meals and snacks more mindfully. In addition, they would participate in and enjoy physical activity as a family. Jake would be encouraged by his parents to try new sports and independently select one that he enjoys. He would learn assertiveness and communication skills so he could effectively manage issues with his peers and learn organizational skills so that he could gain the necessary knowledge and confidence to carry out his healthful goals.

EXERCISE: Building Self-Efficacy

First, show your child the examples of Nora and Jake and explain the concepts, then complete the exercise. He can fill it out independently or collaboratively with you.

What is your core belief(s) about lovability, adequacy, and helplessness? _____

What is your "story?" Are there family dynamics in regard to eating and exercise that reinforce or perpetuate these core beliefs? If yes, how?

_____

_____

What thoughts, feelings, and behaviors are affected based on the core belief(s)?_____

_____

_____

Thoughts: _____

_____

_____

Feelings: _____

_____

_____

Behaviors: _____

_____

_____

How can you build confidence and self-efficacy? _____

_____

_____

When assessing healthy behavior, your child's core beliefs and self-efficacy are strong determinants in predicting his level of success.[70] If you and your child are able to gain an understanding about his self-defeating core beliefs, you can point out when these beliefs are being evoked, predict how they will affect his behavior, and make a conscious effort to change behavior so that it is more healthful. You and your child can also take action to build his self-efficacy and self-confidence.

This exercise can open up a powerful dialogue with your child. You'll get a sense of how he perceives his story and how he thinks that story affects him daily. By helping him be aware of these self-concepts, shift his behavior in response to them, and be more accepting of and generous to himself, he is more likely to take on challenges and stick with a plan. The following strategies point out various family dynamics that affect core beliefs and self-efficacy and provide you with strategies to work through challenges.

R-E-S-P-E-C-T

Convey Mutual Respect and Acceptance

An open relationship with your child is built on mutual respect, genuine understanding, and acceptance of her identity. Particularly if she's over-weight or obese, she'll want to feel that she has *some* control in her life. She may feel that she can't control her weight, eating, and/or fitness behaviors.

Your overall thinking may be, "I'm the parent, so I get to decide on the rules and how I want to carry them out." You might further think, "My child should listen to me because I have more life experience and know what's best for her." While all of that might be fundamentally true, each child is different, and there is no cookie-cutter approach to apply across your household.

If you relentlessly bark demands at her and tell her what she should do about her eating and weight, she is naturally going to resist. She'll take it as you passing judgment on her and believe that you do not think she is capable of thinking independently. In a study where parents as well as children were surveyed, the more frequently parents made comments to their children about their children's weight, the more negatively the children felt about their bodies.[71]

Besides the direct demands that are made of her, your child will also be exposed to expectations or requests regarding her behavior, such as being told to "be sure to eat everything on your plate." Or she may observe you having a piece of cake at a party and then not eating anything the next day aside from drinking coffee in the morning and afternoon. These factors influence her impressions of how she *should* look, feel, and behave in regard to food and her health.

If her perceptions are that your expectations are high and that she most likely won't be able to live up to them, she'll think she should just give up before ever really trying or putting the necessary effort into achieving her healthful goals. She'll expect that failure is inevitable and want to avoid disappointment.

If she feels she can't live up to the family's standards, it can affect her self-confidence and self-compassion and make her feel less valuable—all of which will shape how she behaves. If she is convinced that others view her body negatively, she can become unnecessarily preoccupied with her weight.

120

Keep in mind, these messages are cumulative. They're repeated in different ways at different times. That's why her perceptions, opinions, and judgments get so strongly formed and can stay the same (repeated messages) or change over time (opposing messages from external influences, gaining knowledge, etc.), depending on what she is exposed to.

When you dictate rather than listen to your child express her thoughts, feelings, and needs, you may be missing out on getting to know her on a deep emotional level. Remind yourself that your own thoughts and feelings may affect your desire or willingness to readily listen. Though we cannot control thoughts and feelings, even if we try to, we can control how we react to them.

She knows best what she wants for herself, because she has a good sense of her preferences and what feels right to her. Her feedback is invaluable to you. *The general rule is that your role should be more like that of a coach than a police officer. Kids don't like to be controlled; they prefer to be guided.* It is also best not to micromanage her. Watching every bite that goes into her mouth will make her feel policed and convey that you think that she can't be trusted.

It is essential to practice conveying acceptance and confidence in her abilities, even though you may not appreciate her current behaviors. For example, you're at a friend's house with your child, and she keeps coming back to grab just one more chip, and you are tempted to halt the behavior on the spot and tell her directly to stop. Instead, wait and let the realization come to her on its own, even though she is having more chips than you think she should.

Then, when you have her alone and after you assess that she could be open to hearing you, you say, "I saw you made the choice to keep coming back for more chips and then stopped after a bit. You took the time to think about how you wanted to handle that situation. I'm proud that you considered your values and what you really wanted. This is a practice that you will continue to improve on. I'm here to support and help you if you need me." In this way, you are encouraging her and reinforcing positive behaviors. This will help her focus on moving forward and pushing past the constant insecurity she may be feeling.

Be her coach and ally. You can accomplish that by *asking her opinion, listening to her feedback intently, and proactively involving her in the decision making.* Your dialogue can follow this string. For example, you ask, "What types of exercise would you want to participate in?" After she responds, you mirror back, "I hear that you would be interested in Zumba and

121

kickboxing classes. Do you know of any gyms or facilities that offer them? If not, let's go on the Web together and search for some. I would be happy to join you, or, if you prefer, you can invite a friend to come along." Allowing her to be a part of the decision will make her feel respected, valued, and fundamental to the process. This will result in an increase in her commitment, investment, and ongoing practice of healthful behaviors.

STRATEGY 30

HIDE AND SNEAK

What to Do When Kids and Teens Eat Food in Secret

In my research, many parents reported that their overweight kids "hid" food. Some parents even referred to their children as "stealing" food. The terminology is worth noting, because the way in which you label and think about your child's behavior will directly impact how you approach and deal with his behavior.

Stealing connotes a criminal act and that your child is a thief. If you see him this way, you will more than likely negatively judge, place blame, and punish him for his behavior. This will most likely adversely affect your relationship with him and be a detriment to his self-confidence. If there is food in the house and it is accessible to him, it can never be stealing. He is entitled to any foods that any other family member in the household is entitled to. If it is in the house, it is fair game for all to eat and enjoy. If there are foods that you would prefer your child not eat, make it a point not to have them in your house. For example, you could choose to eliminate ice cream from the house and instead get frozen yogurt, or limit ice cream to one day on the weekend.

Parents often confuse deliberately hiding foods with simply eating alone. Kids I work with often express that they were accused of hiding food when, in their perception, they were not. If your child is leaving empty bowls or wrappers lying around in plain sight, even in his room, where he may not be permitted to eat, he is not hiding food. Hiding takes place when you find empty bowls or wrappers in such areas as behind the couch, under his bed, or otherwise tucked away from plain sight.

Why would he be hiding food, and how should you handle it? Reasons he may be hiding food include:

- he is hungry; perhaps he is going through a growth spurt, is not getting enough calories or fat in his diet, or is burning through most of his calories with physical activities
- he feels deprived of certain foods
- he sees these foods as "forbidden fruit," which he knows you will disapprove of him eating, but he wants them anyway (exerting control and/or independence)
- he uses food for coping (emotional eating)
- he is ashamed that he cannot control his impulses and urges.

The hiding behavior is acted out in secret because of the underlining shame it evokes. He perceives that he "shouldn't" be behaving this way, that his actions are "wrong" and/or "bad," or that his actions will be met with disapproval and possibly harsh consequences. The shame can be self-focused or relative to you. Kids in my research study expressed feeling intense levels of shame when hiding food from their parents. Some sentiments conveying this were, "What's wrong with me? Why can't I control myself?" "My parents will be disappointed with me," or "I know this isn't a healthy choice, so why do I still eat it, anyway?"

When working through this with him, *avoid being reactive and instead deal with the hiding and sneaking behavior separately from the food and eating issues. Pay attention to the act and behavior of hiding, rather than what he's hiding.* The book *How to Get Your Kid to Eat, But Not Too Much* by Ellyn Satter, RD, follows the philosophy that all foods have their place and are best eaten in moderation. With that approach, the message that you're conveying is that all foods are okay, if eaten in moderation. The hiding, secrets, and shame that go along with eating these foods need to be addressed because of the potential barriers they create to a positive, open relationship with himself, you, and food in general.

At the outset, when you begin talking about the hiding with him, if you observe that he is looking away, not maintaining eye contact, or slouching, or he is stammering, speaking softly, or sounds irritated or angry, acknowledge how hard it is to talk about feelings and behavior. Let him know that you are there to listen and understand him better, not to judge him or his behavior.

Also, be sure not to speak in the heat of the moment when you or he may not be up to it. Select an opportunity when you both can actively listen to one another. Last, be sure it isn't a one-sided interrogation without breaks to discuss and reflect on the questions. That can make him feel judged, overwhelmed, and disoriented, which will take away from an open, thoughtful dialogue between the two of you.

Discussion around food hiding should be open-ended, collaborative, and supportive in nature. Focus on the following questions and ideas:

1. Explore in general what he thinks and feels when he is hiding food. You can ask, "What went through your mind when you were hiding the _____?" "How were you feeling about hiding and eating it?" "What was going through your mind after you ate it?" "How did you feel about it?"

2. Why is he hiding the food (as opposed to eating it out in the open)? If he can't readily identify why he's hiding the food even after you prompt him, you can be more direct and offer up the reasons previously mentioned or ask if there is another reason.

3. Ask if he's hungry when he secretly eats, if he feels that there may be something getting in the way of him eating healthy foods, and whether he feels he has access to healthy, nourishing foods. Also check in to see if he can name healthy foods.

4. Investigate whether he feels deprived of certain foods and what specifically is making him feel that way (e.g., his sibling is allowed to eat foods that he's not offered or permitted to eat).

5. Find out if he feels some foods are "forbidden foods" (which make them "good" or "bad") or have rigid "restrictions" on them. How foods are being labeled by family members in his household or outside the home may have an impact on him hiding food (e.g., never have chocolate because it is bad for you, chips are junk food, etc.). Stick to the notion that all food choices are fine in moderation and do not need to be lectured on, worried over, or obsessed about. Stress that food is what the body needs to grow, develop, and sustain itself.

6. Question whether he senses a power struggle between you and him developing and if he wants some more freedom to control what he is and is not eating. You can ask how he would see this independence being created, and develop a concrete plan together (for example, him coming up with a meal plan for several dinners during the week). You could vary his level of freedom and input depending on his age and maturity. While always deciding on a plan collaboratively with him, the younger he is (around the ages of ten to

fourteen), the more you would be direct and offer solutions upfront, because he will probably need more support from you.

7. What does he feel ashamed or embarrassed about, and who he is trying to hide the eating from? You can explore what the particular challenge may be, whether it is emotionally based (see Chapter 4 on HALT) or impulsive and he feels he does not have any control over it, or something else. Explore who specifically he is hiding the eating behavior from (it could be one or both parents, a sibling, all members of the family, etc.) and what he predicts they may be thinking about him based on his eating. Based on his responses, you can address the challenges directly and offer support, reassurance, and the sentiment that he is loved unconditionally, wholeheartedly, and without judgment.

Other practical tips that may help is to not overbuy trigger or craving-inducing foods or keep them in the house. Those are going to be the foods that your child will most likely try to hide. Also, try to "neutralize" the food that he's hiding. Give it to him on a periodic basis so he will no longer feel it's forbidden or overly restricted. When he has access to it regularly, it will lose its luster.

STRATEGY 31

TEAMWORK

Make Change at the Family Level

Change starts at home. I believe in the approach of the family working as a team, because the sum of their concerted effort is more powerful than individual effort. When you shift the focus to the family, together the unit is seeking to improve the family's overall health at the mind-body level. Research shows that children are more successful when the family attempts weight loss and healthier lifestyles together.[72]

Be careful not to push too hard or create too many strict rules around food. Progressively and thoughtfully make changes. If not, you can undermine the family plan and create a situation where goals can't be effectively reached. Then the very food rules that were created to help the family eat more healthily can be the same rules that undermine the practice and leave members craving, feeling deprived, and overeating. Your efforts may be counterproductive.

Even though you may have only one child at home who is overweight or obese, do not single out that child as the one needing improvements to her eating and fitness behaviors. Be sure not to single her out by your actions (such as giving her sibling dessert and not her) or how you communicate (such as comparing her to her thinner sibling). Otherwise, she is likely to feel criticized, ostracized, and punished. These feelings will make her less likely to be motivated to strive for a healthier way of living. Everyone in the family will benefit if the practices are set up thoughtfully and collaboratively. Inevitably, you'll have your own thoughts and feelings about your child's behaviors. Effectively communicating with her will be elaborated on in Chapter 7.

Your child will, of course, ask why you decided to create this change. Answer honestly and candidly that, just like her, you're learning more about health and a healthy lifestyle. Additionally, convey that if she has questions, you'll seek answers to the best of your ability and that you are there to listen and support the family. Here are ways to engage the whole family in the practice.

- Set SMART goals—**S**pecific, **M**easurable, **A**ction-Oriented, **R**ealistic, and **T**ime-Based—so that everyone can participate in them. It's important to start small so that everyone stays committed and feels that they're successfully accomplishing their goals. This can include the family taking a mile walk with the dog three times per week, eating a vegetable at every meal, and/or drinking water instead of juice or soft drinks at meals. Each person can creatively make their own chart such as the one below to illustrate their commitment to the practice.

MY SMART GOAL

- When healthy lifestyles start to become habits, continue to set new goals and aspirations for your family to keep things fun, engaging, and rewarding. For example, make hikes longer and more challenging, and vary locations by traveling different scenic routes.

- If it used to be customary to go out to eat for special occasions, celebrate a family milestone by cooking a healthy recipe together instead. Eating out is costly, portion sizes tend to be large, and we do not know what ingredients are in our food. There could be added preservatives, dyes, excessive amounts of oil and butter, etc., that we are not aware of. Try to eat out less often and cook at home. When you do decide to eat out, encourage your children to assert their health needs, such as asking servers to eliminate butter and margarine from foods or to go light on the oil.

- Many added sugar calories are eaten at home.[73] This can be monitored and prevented. For example, for dessert, decide on fresh fruit, such as watermelon, mango, or pineapple, all-fruit ice pops, or angel food cake with baked fruit or a bit of fruit sorbet. Also, always have fruits and vegetables on hand.

- Go shopping for healthy ingredients, select recipes, and prepare meals together (see Resources for a variety of family cookbooks). For example, you could choose to cook several meals together and rotate which person plans the menu, or create a culinary challenge to see who can create the healthiest and tastiest meal. You could pair up younger children with an older sibling or parent and rotate teams, as well. There are numerous studies showing the direct correlation between family meals and health.[74] When families eat meals together, kids tend to eat healthier and are less likely to be overweight.

- Before you shop, take an inventory of what each individual's preferences are (fruit, vegetables, etc.), what trigger foods not to buy or have around your house, and what healthy snacks everyone can agree on. Make sure to always have healthy snacks readily available at home.

- Plan your shopping trips so that they aren't during a time of day when family members are especially hungry or have cravings, so that purchases are thought through rather than motivated by impulse.

- When talking about food, avoid demonizing and/or glorifying food of any kind. Family members should avoid using derogatory labels for food such as "junk" or "bad" food, which can perpetuate feelings of guilt and shame. Also, candy and sweets shouldn't be glorified as the most sought-after foods. All foods should be considered for both pleasure and sustenance and appreciated for what they offer.

- Don't use food as rewards or punishments. Family members should decide together to use alternatives for rewards, such as spending time with each other or participating in an activity together. If children perceive parents as withholding or taking away food, they may fear hunger or overeat at a later point in time.
- Make a commitment to learn how to be more healthful as a family. For example, during Sunday family meeting night, you could look up varying ways to engage in family activities, the risks of heart disease, and facts about nutrition.
- Make rules about where food can be eaten, and designate eating areas in your home. Make the rules for the house, not singling out any particular child.
- Many studies found a direct correlation between screen time and kids being overweight and obese.[75] As a family, commit to no more than two hours of screen time a day. This is a direct recommendation from the American Academy of Pediatrics.[76]
- To reinforce mindful eating practices, as a family rule, commit to screen-free mealtimes.
- Consider outfitting each member of the family with a pedometer or activity tracker to encourage healthy habits. You can chart progress, check on your SMART goals, and institute new ones as warranted.
- Institute healthy sleeping habits. According to the National Sleep Foundation, five- to twelve-year-olds need ten to eleven hours of sleep a day, and twelve- to eighteen-year-olds need at least eight and a half hours per day.[77] Research shows that there is a direct correlation between poor sleeping habits and weight gain.[78]

Change has to happen at the family level so that everyone is supporting each other during challenges, triumphs, and moments of adversity. Each member will feel invested in the process and hold each other accountable in a meaningful way. Once the process of working together as a family for good health is in place, it can be used as a template for handling other challenges.

CHECK YOUR BAGGAGE

This chapter focused on how the family can be instrumental in facilitating healthy practices in your household. The intent is not to blame you as a parent or the family as a whole, but rather to empower you to recognize that you are integral to contributing to your child's health.

As parents, we need to set examples for our children and model the behaviors that we hope they will learn. Consistency is key! We have a responsibility to assess ourselves at the core level, as well, and take an inventory of how we think, feel, and behave so that we can be most helpful to our children. We also have the responsibility to create an environment where health is openly talked about, where there's safety in asserting needs, and where individual family members' needs can be addressed. It's our obligation to ensure the health of our children and ourselves.

In this chapter, you were encouraged to examine your actions and pay attention to thoughts and feelings that may influence your child. Check in with yourself. Assess both your and your child's core beliefs and how they affect your and your child's thoughts, feelings, and behaviors. Also, question whether you are effectively practicing mutual respect and partnering in your child's health goals, rather than being demanding or micromanaging.

Consider how you think and feel about your child's specific behaviors, such as hiding food, overeating, emotionally eating, etc. How does that impact your perceptions of your child, how you communicate, and eventually how you behave toward your child? Your child's behaviors will likely evoke thoughts and feelings that you cannot control, but your behavior toward your child is something you can effectively work on.

Working as a team may be a shift in how your family has functioned in the past—consider how you are experiencing that change, as well. With changes, there may be doubt or enthusiasm. Monitor where your family is during different stages of the process, and check in with how you are feeling about it all.

This is a learning experience for you. As long as you are monitoring where you are in the process, accommodating your thoughts and feelings, and being cognizant of how you are behaving, you are doing all that you can to facilitate a positive family dynamic, connection, and mutual support.

 REVIEW

You and your family members are major contributors in facilitating healthful practices in your household. The family functions as a team to carry out the process and practice of good health and wellness.

Parents should continually assess:

- Thoughts
- Feelings
- Ways you communicate on behalf of your thoughts and feelings
- Ways you communicate support and care
- How you take action to facilitate open communication with your child
- Actions/speech
- Family dynamics
- Core beliefs and the strength of your child's self-efficacy
- Whether you are carrying out a relationship with your child based on mutual respect
- If and how you are effectively working through specific challenges as they come up
- Whether you are facilitating a team approach in your household
- If you are taking effective action based on the team approach.

 MINDFULNESS EXERCISE: You Are Who You Are

See page 223 for the mindfulness exercise that corresponds to this chapter, and refer to page 217 for instructions on accessing the audio.

The Many Facets of Communicating

My mother insists I see a nutritionist to help me make healthy food choices. It's nothing I haven't heard before or learned in health class. I don't know why she's wasting her money. I want to do this on my own, but she won't just leave me alone about it. One day it's a new diet, another day a new exercise class. She's a real royal pain.

—BRIANNA, AGE 14

I try to make suggestions to my son about getting in better shape for football season. He let himself slide over the summer, and it's going to affect his game. He's sluggish and out of shape. He constantly tells me I'm criticizing him and gives me an attitude when I raise it. I'm just mentioning it to him because I care, and I want him to be at the top of his game for the upcoming season.   —VICTOR, PARENT

I N THIS CHAPTER, you'll learn how to effectively listen to, communicate with, and support your child in a loving way when it comes to topics such as health and weight. It's all about active listening: how parent and child can organize their thoughts before speaking, practice what they are going to say, and use nonjudgmental language. By conveying trust and empathy, parents show their children that they care about their needs, and the children will be more inclined to express themselves.

For example, let's say your child is waiting to go out to dinner with you in an hour. He says that he's slightly hungry, and he's eyeing the cookies in the cabinet. As a parent, you know if you weren't standing right there, he would go straight for the cookies, no questions asked. You can't help but think to yourself, *We're going out in an hour; why can't he just wait? We just had lunch a couple of hours ago. It's so frustrating that he has no self-control and thinks so much about eating sweets.* With those thoughts bouncing around in your head, you want to say: "You just ate! We're going out soon. Can't you just wait? I always have to tell you to watch yourself! Can't you think about it yourself?" These statements are full of judgment and criticism, and, if you combine that with an annoyed tone, he'll definitely pick up on your disapproval of him.

After working through this chapter, you will learn to let go of that first impulse and speak in a way that's more mindful and productive. Instead of sounding critical, you might say, "I get that you're feeling hungry and that it's still a while until dinner. It's hard to wait when we want something. When we're hungry, truly physically hungry, we aren't selective about we eat. Maybe this is just a craving, which I totally get, because I get them all the time, too. I know you want the cookies, but do you think you could be mindful and choose something healthier that could get you through until dinner? It's your choice, and I know you want to make a good one, because it's important to you."

By utilizing the elements of good communication, which include normalizing impulses, acknowledging feelings, pointing out alternatives, and gently reminding your child of his goals and core values, this situation becomes much less tense.

If he opens up about his cravings, he might say something like, "I wish I thought and felt differently" or, "I can't stand the way I think sometimes; I worry that I'll never be successful at this." Using refined communications skills, you can offer further support by actively listening to his concerns and expressing to him that thoughts are *not* automatically facts ("I must have the cookies")—they are only so if he makes them facts. He has the power to adjust his actions and decide how he wants to behave.

Take the time, effort, and patience to gently work with your child. Though you may not always like what he is saying, it's still important to communicate acceptance of and openness to what he thinks and feels, especially about difficult topics such as food, health, and weight. Even if it is hard at first, demonstrating honesty and a willingness to listen without judging is the hallmark of an open, communicative relationship with your child.

GET IN TOUCH

Tap into Thoughts and Feelings on Food, Weight, and Health

As a parent, you are responsible for being aware of your own thoughts, feelings, and judgments and for acting in your child's best interest. As previously noted, whatever feelings and thoughts come up for you are also okay. You get to choose how and if you want to act on those thoughts and feelings.

Parents may demonstrate weight bias toward their children.[79] A study on parents' perceptions of health professionals' responses when seeking help for their overweight children showed that parents often feel stigmatized or blamed (that they are bad parents and are neglecting their children, aren't teaching them well, are passing down the genes to them, etc.).[80] These factors can directly affect how they communicate with and act toward their children.[81]

Nearly half of mothers and a third of fathers have been reported to show weight bias.[82] Surprisingly, fathers with higher education and income were more likely to endorse stereotypes, as were both parents who reported a strong investment in their own appearance. Also, parents who were overweight and obese were just as likely to endorse stereotypes as thinner parents.[83] These statistics highlight how we are all vulnerable to biases and need to be aware of them.

You may have your own biases and feelings of frustration or anger when it comes to your child's weight. Our culture helps shape and perpetuate those feelings. So, if you're thinking and feeling that way, know that you are most definitely not alone.

Being conscientious and self-aware of these thoughts and feelings is the first step at working through them for the benefit of you and your child. Even if you feel these feelings, you can still make it a point to communicate openly, empathize with your child, and care for her.

Even with open communication, unwelcome feelings may come up when you talk to her about her weight and health. These topics may be uncomfortable for you for many reasons. Perhaps they were taboo in your own family growing up, you are not sure how to talk about them, and/or you don't feel savvy enough to talk about the topic because you have been grappling with your own weight challenges.

Despite this, you still need to make a commitment and be willing to talk about anything that comes up for you and her. Just as it's critical to talk about drugs, sex, and Internet safety with her, it is equally important to speak about eating behaviors and exercising. These are not issues she'll just outgrow; obesity puts her health at risk.

Some topics that you can expect to come up include eating disorders, "junk" food, body image, self-perception, the "F" word ("fat"), etc. To open a dialogue with her, you may consider asking her how she feels about her body. Does she think about it often? Are there specific pressures that she feels regarding her eating behaviors and fitness? You may also use the questions that follow in this chapter to help structure your discussion with her.

Remember, nothing is off-limits. Your child needs to feel that there is safety in communicating with you at any time about anything. If she doesn't bring it up to you, you are not off the hook. It is your responsibility to raise the issue with her—particularly if you sense that the topic is troubling her or affecting her negatively in any way.

The majority of parents I interviewed said that they were concerned that if they spoke with their children about their children's challenges with their eating and exercise behaviors, they were going to say or do the wrong thing and hurt them, put thoughts in their mind, or create an eating disorder for their children.

If your child is overweight or obese, you can guarantee that she knows it. Her mirror broadcasts it, she may be teased at school or by her siblings, and/or she's observing enough images on television and in magazines about how she's "supposed" to look. By not saying something, you are making a choice to ignore the obvious, which can result in her feeling isolated and alone with her frustration and pain. She may be left with her own set of judgments about the way you and others perceive her.

If you take the time to open up dialogue in a caring and nurturing way, it will give you the ability to provide her with knowledge, clarification, comfort, and reassurance, which is what every kid needs and is entitled to. If she is thinking about or engaging in some method of disordered eating, she will be more open to seeking support if you start a dialogue.

In my research, many parents reported feelings of guilt, anger, frustration, and hopelessness because they did not know how to successfully help their children improve their health. You are not expected to know how off the bat, but you can learn the skills to be helpful to your child. The sooner you bring up the challenges, the better. While it is possible at any age, it is much easier to tackle health issues when a child is younger and more open to making changes. Also, keep in mind that overweight or obese children are ten times more likely to become overweight or obese adults.[84] This sets them up for serious health concerns in adulthood.[85]

Studies show that it is not only important and essential that parents speak about health and body image with their children, but attention also needs to be paid to *how* you speak about them in order to increase healthful eating behaviors.[86] You also have your own relationship with food and health that is bound to be evoked when you're dealing with your child's issues. If you have or had a tenuous relationship with food and your health, those thoughts and feelings are likely to seep in.

With groups of parents I have met, many expressed feelings of shame and embarrassment. They felt their children's challenges signified a lack of the family's ability to have self-discipline, which in turn was a reflection of them and their lack of control. For those parents who were particularly challenged with impulsiveness, perfectionism, or rigidity much of the time, when their children engaged in overeating, it triggered in the adults feelings of frustration, disappointment, and fear. Derived from our personal challenges, we often make conscious or unconscious rules in our minds, which influences how we see the world, how we perceive ourselves, and how family members "ought" to be.

EXERCISE: Consider Your Own History with Eating and Exercising

You may instinctively think that your child "should," "must," and "ought to" behave in certain ways, and when she is not in sync with those expectations, you become angry and frustrated with her. Ask yourself these questions to gain perspective on how your own history with food may evoke these feelings about yourself and your child.

- What was your relationship with food as a child and growing up? Do you consider it a generally negative or positive one? For example, were you preoccupied with or did you struggle with thoughts about food, eating, weight, or fitness?
- Did your parents and family model healthful eating and exercise behaviors?
- What *explicit* (straightforward, directly communicated) messages did you get from your parents or family regarding food, eating, weight, and fitness?
- What *implicit* messages (such as body language or what wasn't

said but was understood) did you get from your parents or family regarding food, eating, weight, and fitness?

- How did these explicit and implicit messages affect you in regard to your thinking and behavior?
- What explicit and implicit messages did you receive from the outside world (friends, media, etc.) regarding food, eating, weight, and fitness?
- How did these messages affect you in regard to your thinking and behavior?
- Did you have access to knowledge regarding healthy eating and exercising?
- Where did you obtain this knowledge? Was it accurate information?
- How did you feel about your eating, weight, and exercise behavior?
- Did that change over time? How? Why?
- Growing up, how did you feel about your body?
- Did that change over time? How? Why?
- Were you ever picked on or teased about your weight, eating, or fitness behaviors? If yes, by whom? How did you experience it? How did it affect you?

It is important to gain perspective on the feelings that you tap into when you and your child talk about eating or exercise behaviors. Yes, it is "when" and not "if" these feelings get tapped into, because it is very likely to happen. If you are in touch with those triggers, you will be prepared and can be more mindful about how you behave toward your child.

STRATEGY 33

YOUR BODY SPEAKS, TOO

Communication Dos and Don'ts

How we communicate, both directly (through speech) and indirectly (through body language), conveys our judgments and expectations. Whether we say something out loud or just grimace, kids read us loudly and clearly. Assess your direct and indirect communication patterns; both patterns are equally important and impactful.

Kids forever remember when they first heard that they are "fat," "chubby," or "overweight." As much as you would like to protect them from the labels that cause them to question their own self-worth, you can't always protect them from other people. You can only make sure the messages *you* communicate (through words and behaviors) do not convey judgment, disappointment, or disdain.

As a parent, it is essential for you to convey acceptance of your child without any contingencies. In a large study of adolescents and their parents, scientists examined the correlation between parental conversations about healthful eating and weight and disordered eating behaviors in adolescents. The study showed that parents who engaged in *weight-related* conversations had adolescents who were more likely to diet, use unhealthy weight-control behaviors, and engage in binge eating. Adolescents whose parents engaged in conversations that were focused only on *healthful eating behaviors* were less likely to diet and use unhealthy weight-control behaviors.[87]

In the study, the weight-related conversations included discussion of their children's weight and size. Parents conveyed to their children that they were heavy or were going to get fat if they continued to eat the way they did. The results clearly indicate that children used desperate, unhealthy, and often dangerous methods to "work on" their challenge because of feeling that their parents would be more approving and accepting of them and love them more if they were thinner.

Kids often hide away during adolescence; they are trying to form their identity. They seek independence and autonomy balanced with a sense of belonging and feeling they are approved of.

Never shame your child or call him names. Even though you may mean it playfully, he may not take it that way. Teasing isn't positive unless both parties perceive it as fun. That's often not the case. The teasers perceive it as lighthearted and fun, while those teased often describe the same situation as malicious and irritating.[88]

Calling him "chubby cheeks" or "muffin top" may sound cute but can be quite damaging to a child's confidence. Parents who approach weight in counterproductive ways, such as teasing, put children at higher risk for developing disordered eating behaviors such as anorexia, bulimia, and binge eating.[89] It also puts young women at risk for selecting romantic partners who make hurtful comments about their weight.[90] They internalize the teasing; they think they are deserving of it and should expect it from those who are close to them.[91] In addition, taking parental modeling into account, if children see their parents participating in teasing, they may think it is permissible, and it gives them free rein to tease others.

BEHAVIORS THAT ARE *NOT* HELPFUL FOR FOSTERING OPEN DIALOGUE:

1. Teasing your child about his weight or body.

2. Badgering your child about his weight and eating habits.

3. Nagging or preaching to your child about what to eat, when to eat, and to eat less than he's eating.

4. Talking to your child about diets.

5. Rewarding or bribing your child to eat differently.

6. Commenting negatively on weight loss or weight gain.

7. Weighing your child.

8. Rejecting him for any changes in his body weight.

A ROAD MAP FOR HAVING OPEN AND ENRICHING DISCUSSIONS:

1. Thanking your child for his willingness to speak to you and for expressing his thoughts and feelings.

2. Being aware of how you are directly and indirectly communicating. Encourage your child with reassuring sentiments ("You can do it" and "You are really putting a lot of effort into this") and warm and supportive body language (smiling and being affectionate).

3. Using empowering terminology when discussing your child's health (e.g., use words such as "healthy," "flexible," "agile," "fit," "strong," and "active").

4. Using open-ended questions to decrease the chance that your child will give you one-word answers, so the discussion can develop.

5. Being sure to listen more than you speak. Parents can get caught up in teaching and lecturing; you run the risk that your child will tune you out because of feeling talked at and bored.

138

6. Hearing your child out fully at the outset; find out what he needs and what he's looking for and expecting from you. Avoid offering advice or solutions prematurely.

7. During the conversation, checking in to be sure you understand what your child is trying to communicate to you. You can effectively accomplish this by paraphrasing (restating in your own words), summarizing (summing up concisely), and mirroring (reflecting back verbatim) what he says.

8. Always offering to collaborate and work together as a team. The more support your child receives, the greater the chance that he will be open to talking about this topic, ask for help when he needs it, and put effort into making changes.

9. Keeping the conversation open. Let your child know you will always be available to speak to him and that there's an open-door policy regarding communication.

10. Respecting when your child doesn't want to speak and letting him know that you're around when he's ready to open up.

11. Normalizing the challenges. Convey that kids can face a variety of health challenges—asthma or allergies, for example—and that challenges do not define who they are or their potential for success.

STRATEGY 34

SHOWING EMPATHY

Communicate Support and Unconditional Love

In our popular media, being thin is desirable and the seeming definition of "beauty." This can be demoralizing for your child. You obviously won't be able to completely counter these influences; however, you can emphasize what's important. The key with communicating is conveying empathy: overall acceptance, care, and unconditional love. This should consistently be the underlying theme.

Communicate to your child that:

- Before and after puberty, our bodies change dramatically, and weight gain can be a normal part of the process.

- Healthy behavior is important because it helps our bodies grow, function properly, and become strong.
- By engaging in healthful behaviors, she is helping her body stay energetic, not overwork her organs (such as the heart, lungs, etc.), and avoid injury.
- Part of loving herself means taking care of her body and keeping it strong and healthy by eating healthfully and exercising.
- Our appearance does not determine our worth.
- Physical attributes in general do not determine our worth. Her worth to you is not determined by her shape or size or what she looks like.
- How much she weighs is not a measure of who she is as a person. Who she is (a caring friend, a conscientious student, etc.) is the true measure of her as a person.
- You have unconditional love for her.
- You would love her just as much if she looked different and had, for example, a different height or hair color or was heavier or thinner.
- Our body size and shape are in part due to heredity, much the same as eye color and height.
- You appreciate diversity and differences. Emphasize to your child that her size and shape contribute to her uniqueness. Uniqueness contributes to her individual beauty. You can use examples such as fish and flowers, which come in different shapes, sizes, and colors. Stress that each is special in its own way.
- She is taking positive action toward her health by doing _____. (Avoid focusing on all that she may not be doing).
- There are challenges to being and staying healthy (you can relay your own), but the benefits of better health are worth the time and effort you put into it.
- What is truly important to you is the effort, rather than the results, and that you are proud of her commitment made toward her health.

Even with all that you are going to say to her, you will undoubtedly hear concern from her about her body. For example, a typical question is

"Does this make me look fat?" Our inclination is to respond directly to what she is asking, reassure her how wonderful and beautiful she is, and convince her that how she looks is not something she should "worry about," is "not important," and should "not be her central focus."

I assume you have done this before. We all have! Good luck trying to convince her. That is where her mind is, given her stage of development. She tends to hyper-focus on her social stature, others' perceptions of her, and the way she looks. That is appropriate for girls and boys of her age, and the degree of concern varies from teen to teen. We have to meet kids and teens where they are. We have to ensure that we're making meaningful effort to "get" or understand our children.

Rather than responding quickly and directly to the question, make it a point to understand where she is coming from and what meaning the question holds for her. By doing so, you can develop both a deeper level of understanding of her challenges and empathy for her. Mirror (reflect back) to her what you heard. For example, you can say, "I heard you ask me if you look fat. Can you please tell me what you're concerned about if you *were* to look fat? I'm interested in hearing more about your concerns." After fully hearing her out, you can acknowledge and empathize with her concerns and return to the sentiments mentioned earlier.

When you respond in an empathic way, you're showing interest in her. It shows your child that you want to learn more about how she thinks and feels and that you are actually hearing and taking in what she says. This care goes a long way in helping to forge self-confidence, self-compassion, and self-awareness within her.

NOT CUT FROM THE SAME CLOTH

Handle Sibling Teasing

The old sentiment about family is that we are all "cut from the same cloth." But as you may have experienced, although you share similar genes, you may be very different from your parents or siblings—sometimes so much so that you question whether you belong to that family. Body type is a characteristic that often varies from person to person within the same family.

In my research, parents often reported that a typical challenge is how to handle it when one of their children is of average weight and the other is overweight or obese. This creates confusion around serving food and how to handle weight teasing among siblings. We tackle this food issue (see page 125) by creating equanimity across the family and presenting a family lifestyle shift for all. This minimizes resentment in your overeating child and could prevent your other children from feeling they have permission to be hurtful or cruel toward their sibling.

Parents expressed being distressed over name-calling and weight shaming that they directly observed or heard about from one of their children. Weight-based teasing by family members is extremely common. Nearly half of overweight females and a third of overweight males reported experiencing weight-based teasing by family members.[92] Although it's common and most often demonstrated by brothers toward their sisters,[93] it also occurs among same-gender siblings and sisters toward their brothers. Teasing in general comes with emotional detriments and is associated with a higher BMI in the affected child in the long term.[94]

Parents participating in my research were at a loss about how to address such teasing with their children. As a result, most reported that they did not say anything, in the hope that their children would work it out among themselves. Some came to the rescue of the victim and expressed belligerence toward their other children for being so cruel, and others tried to remain neutral and just expressed how weight and fat shaming was not acceptable in their household. As a parent, would you know how to handle this type of teasing behavior?

HOW TO HANDLE WEIGHT-BASED TEASING AMONG SIBLINGS

1. In your household, foster a cooperative and supportive sibling spirit, rather than a competitive, resentful one. This entails being conscious of not comparing one child to the other, showing preferences, siding with one or the other, etc. The book *Siblings Without Rivalry: How to Help Your Children Live Together So You Can Live Too* by Adele Faber and Elaine Mazlish masterfully points out strategic ways to effectively manage sibling relationships.

2. Have a no-tolerance policy regarding teasing in your household, and be sure to stick to it. Convey that kids need to express what behavior they are being frustrated by, not put down or label their sibling or anyone else.

142

3. When they do tease, put the focus on the teasing (the behavior), not the content of the teasing (such as weight). Acknowledge the feeling behind the teasing, but don't give credence to the remark. Make it a house rule that when family members want to express anger, frustration, agitation, etc., they need to do it in a productive way to foster communication, understanding, and effective action.

   For example, let's say your son says to your daughter, "You're such a fat pig." First, *acknowledge his feelings*: "You sound really angry." Second, *remind him of this rule*: "What you said was out of sync with our family rule of not being hurtful to each other by teasing or insulting." Third, *remind him that he needs to express his thoughts and feelings in a helpful way*: "I want to hear what you have to say. Can you share how you feel about your sister's behavior so that she can understand you better?" He might respond, "When you ate an additional popsicle, it didn't leave any for me, and I am feeling frustrated at you because I wanted one, too. Please make sure that we all have one before you take another one."

4. Let kids know that you are only willing to listen to them if they express the feeling rather than the insult. If they persist, ignore them until they are ready to share meaningfully and drop the pejoratives. You can say, "I can't hear what you're saying because you're not following the rules of not insulting or teasing in this house. When you're able to express how you feel about your sister's behavior, I'm happy to listen to you." (Don't say, "You insulted her," because it could be misconstrued that you are taking sides, which would just escalate his anger.)

5. Step in right away if you observe teasing. You are stepping in because your zero-tolerance policy isn't being followed. Make it clear that you are the parent and are responsible for ensuring that the rules of the household are being followed. This action takes away from the possible perception that you're taking sides in the situation and shows that you are being proactive in maintaining mutual respect and integrity in your household.

6. If you are not directly in the crossfire, wait to see if your children can work it out themselves. Observe whether they can independently reboot and get back on track to adhere to the household rules and effectively manage their communication and relationship. This may be a bit more difficult for younger kids or kids who have challenges with impulsivity. In this case you may need to step in more frequently or sooner than you typically would. If the tension noticeably escalates, and they are having a hard time hearing one another, step in.

7. During downtime, such as a family meeting, discuss each family member's challenges, how they feel about it, and how they work on it. Have each member ask the family or select members to support them in specific ways. This neutralizes the issues and stigmatization associated with weight and allows everyone to gain insight and empathy. It also facilitates openness to discussing a challenge, rather than mocking, belittling, or minimizing it by shaming or teasing.

For example, I use the abbreviation **CFWA**: identify the **C**hallenge, identify **F**eelings about it, **W**ork on it, and provide **A**ssistance your children need. Those are the initials of the names of each of my children, so that they remember it. You could creatively find or create your own abbreviation as a family. I also emphasize confidentiality, so all family members respect each other's privacy around a challenge and don't discuss it outside the family unless that person is open to it. We do a review monthly at the family meeting, checking in on how they are feeling and dealing with their challenges and whether they need to amend practices or request further support.

KNOWLEDGE IS POWER

Increase Your Knowledge Base

As a parent, you are not expected to know everything. Assess for yourself how much knowledge you have about nutrition and fitness. If you feel you are knowledgeable and can teach your child the basics, great. But if you find yourself confused by the plethora of information out there or don't feel that you have enough of a knowledge base, you could seek to

FREE YOUR CHILD FROM OVEREATING

learn with your child by researching or by meeting with a nutritionist.

Teach yourself and your child about body diversity and the causes of being overweight or obese. This will help debunk some of the myths that you and he may believe regarding weight and health. Some books that can help with this include *Self-Esteem Comes in All Sizes* by Carol Johnson, *Fat Kids: Truth and Consequences* by Rebecca Jane Weinstein, and *Big Fat Lies* by Glenn Gaesser.

Your child will inevitably feel more empowered if he has the information he needs to make more mindful decisions regarding his eating and exercise behaviors. He, too, may be confused.

Keep in mind that eventually your child will be independent of you and will need to make choices for himself, so you want to educate him as best as you can so that he is fully equipped to make mindful decisions regarding his eating and fitness behaviors. *The goal for any child is to promote diet-free living and mindful eating with all foods eaten in moderation.*

Critical facts you should know and may want to convey to your child (based on age, maturity, and stage of development) include:

1. Diets don't work. Ninety-five percent of all dieters regain their lost weight in one to five years.[95] Diets are often unhealthy and can be counterproductive. Girls who diet frequently are twelve times as likely to binge as girls who don't diet.[96] Encouraging dieting can undermine parents' intent and actually contribute to an increased risk of obesity.[97]

2. In 2013, the American Medical Association officially deemed obesity a disease. That means that a quick fix will not do the trick. A consistent practice of healthy eating and exercise will make long-term, incremental changes.

3. It is helpful to follow the 80/20 rule: Healthy eating can be successfully maintained if it's accomplished 80 percent of the time. There shouldn't be rigidity to eating. Rather, it should encompass balance and moderation.

4. Being overweight or obese can be the result of a complex combination of genetics and environmental and health behaviors, including dietary intake and physical activity.[98]

5. There can be physiological factors that contribute to weight (e.g., thyroid function, hormones, and metabolism).

6. The calories in/calories out approach is a common, oversimplified, and outdated approach. Food is more than the calories it contains, and all calories are not created equal. The type of calories in food are "instructions" to your body to create either health or disease. A diet low in protein results in bad fat being stored around your organs, while high-protein diets add muscle and increase your resting metabolism and muscle mass. That's a good thing, because muscle burns seven times as many calories as fat.[99]

7. Research on high-fat diets shows direct evidence of sustained injury to the part of the brain that helps regulate food intake. A study showed that within three days of being placed on a high-fat diet, a rat's hypothalamus showed increased inflammation. Within a week, there was evidence of permanent scarring and neuron injury in the area of the brain that is crucial for weight control. Brain scans of obese men and women show the same pattern.[100]

8. Research shows that 90 percent of the dopamine receptors in the reward center of the brain are activated in response to food cues. This compels us to want more and more hyper-palatable foods.[101] These are foods layered in salt, fat, and sweet flavors, which are all proven to increase consumption when we eat them. Food manufacturers know this and use it to keep you and your children hooked.

9. Studies have proven that food can be addictive. That's why people binge on potato chips, chocolate, or cupcakes more often than on carrot sticks and apple slices. Brain imaging using PET scans showed that high-sugar and high-fat foods work just like drugs such as heroin, opium, or morphine. People also develop a tolerance of sugar; they will need more and more to get satisfied.[102]

10. Research shows that, when given a choice, rats were more attracted to sweetened water than to cocaine or heroin.[103] As for your biochemistry, when you consume glucose, a type of sugar, it spikes your blood sugar and causes high insulin levels. High insulin then blocks leptin, your appetite hormone, so your brain doesn't get the "I'm full" signal and instead thinks you're starving.

Your pleasure-based reward center becomes activated, which drives you to consume more sugar. This explains why your child may have difficulty controlling the consumption of foods high in sugar.

11. There is no nutritional value in "added" sugar. This refers to the sugar that is added to food during processing (e.g., sucrose, fructose, etc.). It contains no protein, vitamins, minerals, or fiber. Even though the American Heart Association recommends no more than 3 teaspoons (12 grams) of added sugar per day for kids, according to the National Health and Nutrition Examination Survey administered by the CDC, boys are consuming on average 23 teaspoons and girls 18 teaspoons per day.[104] If your child drinks a 20-ounce bottle of original Gatorade, he would have consumed three times his sugar allowance for the day.

12. Overeating is learned and becomes a habit. We are triggered (see the enticing food), engage in eating behavior, and then get rewarded by the behavior (experience pleasure because it tastes so incredibly good, feel better emotionally, etc.). We commit to memory the reward process and continually chase that pleasure (the first delicious bite, the immediate joyfulness, etc.). This is why it feels like it's so difficult to change the behavior, because it's what we have learned and what has become engrained in our memory. We naturally make these associations when we eat. (Listen to Judson Brewer's TED Talk "A Simple Way to Break a Bad Habit" to learn why mindfulness is helpful with this process and refer to page 110 for how long it takes to change or develop new habits.)

Check in with your child. Ask him the following questions to establish how you can best help him obtain helpful knowledge about nutrition:

- Do you feel you have the knowledge you need in order to eat nutritiously and healthfully?
- Do you feel you have the knowledge you need in order to participate in physical fitness?
- Where did you receive this knowledge?
- Is any of the information regarding nutrition or fitness confusing to you?

- How can I best help you to obtain this knowledge? Would you prefer me to teach you or do you prefer meeting with a nutritionist to learn this information?

Notice the last question was not about whether he should or should not learn, but *how* he would learn. As a parent, you do not have to teach it to him yourself, particularly if you do not feel that you are equipped to, but you do have the responsibility to provide him with the resources (a nutritionist, holistic health coach, physician, etc.) so that he can successfully acquire the knowledge.

 ## CHECK YOUR BAGGAGE

As a parent, you are responsible for being aware of how your thoughts and feelings affect your communication. We all have personal histories that shape our perceptions of our weight and health. Consider your history and how it directly affects your willingness to talk with your child. Speaking about topics such as eating and exercise is typically not an easy task but one we choose to do because we must.

Check in with yourself and assess your direct and indirect methods of communicating:

- Are you conveying empathy, encouragement, care, and unconditional love? Or dismay, dissatisfaction, and frustration?

- Are there barriers that get in the way of open and enriching dialogue and communication with your child? Are you seeking to work through those and implement more effective methods?

- When you are communicating support, does it feel genuine? If it does not, what are some ways you could connect with your child more effectively?

- How knowledgeable are you about healthful eating? What resources do you need to acquire additional knowledge?

 ## REVIEW

Effectively communicating with your child is critical. You may never have been taught this and are not expected to know how to right away. With a sensitive topic such as weight, good communication is not always instinctual.

Within one family, there are many individuals who each think, feel, and behave quite differently. Effective communication skills will help you forge a more connected and loving relationship with your child, so that speaking about a challenging topic can be more manageable and satisfying. Here's a summary of what to do to practice effective communication with your child.

Parents can:

- Get in touch with their own thoughts and feelings about their children's weight and health challenges.
- Consider their personal history in relationship to their own weight and health.
- Gain awareness of their own thoughts and feelings about their personal weight and health challenges.
- Assess what strategies they are currently using that may *not* be helpful for fostering open dialogue.
- Evaluate if they are utilizing effective methods of communicating with their children, or if obstacles might be getting in the way.
- Apply effective communication methods if there is teasing between siblings.
- Gain knowledge about healthful eating and behavior and either personally convey it to their children or seek resources so that their children can effectively learn it from a credible source.

 MINDFULNESS EXERCISE: Freedom to Be

See page 224 for the mindfulness exercise that corresponds to this chapter, and refer to page 217 for instructions on accessing the audio.

8

Friends and Other Outside Influences

It's so much pressure to get together with friends. There's so much gossip around who looks good and what everyone is wearing. I sit there and pray that I won't be up for discussion, and they won't notice me.
— DEBRA, AGE 14

I hear the sighs when I'm picked for their team. Do they really need to be so obvious about it? I'm trying to be active and get involved, but it's not very easy when kids are so mean.   — BRETT, AGE 16

WE'VE DISCUSSED THE ROLE of families in children's health, but you can't talk about kids and teens without talking about their friendships. Although parents are a powerful force in their children's lives, peers exert an equally strong pull. Their friends profoundly affect the way kids and teens eat, exercise, and, most important, feel about themselves and their bodies. Some of these influences are positive; however, some are not.

This chapter will show you how to educate your kids about how they are developing and changing: physically, emotionally, and psychologically. Most important, you and they should know that what they are going through is normal and that the trials and tribulations of these years will not last forever. Even though most kids feel confused and alone sometimes, kids struggling with weight and self-confidence issues often feel lonely due to social isolation and the pressure to conform.

In elementary school and sometimes at the beginning of middle school, kids prefer being with their parents, but as the teen years come upon them, family time tends to be history. Friends and social networks are the new priority. When you finally get your child to sit down with you,

you must understand that he is using most of his brainpower to think about school, relationships, etc. Kids and teens often evaluate themselves in terms of how successful they feel in their friendships. If they have close friends, they want to keep them; they want to have an influence on their group. Your child wants to be liked, cared for, and included. Who doesn't?

Sometimes, they may not feel as successful as you (or possibly they) would like and find themselves disappointed, frustrated, and sad. Even those who do have close friends can have mixed feelings about the people they hang out with. Sometimes they are satisfied; other times they are sure others do not "get" them, and they feel shut out. They may wonder, "Will these be my friends for years to come?" When they think of branching out, they wonder, "What would that be like?"

Teens and their friends often experience these confusing emotions at the same time, which can lead to misunderstandings and conflicts. Sometimes they adore their friends, while other times they want to trade them in for a new batch. They feel one way, then the other. Then both! These varying emotions are not only affected by their present circumstance, but also by their mood, their hormones, and how they are feeling about themselves in the moment.

Teens may also have interest in intimate relationships, which further define them and their friendships. They are interested in their friends approving of their relationship choices and spend a great deal of time considering what might happen if they do not. They may like someone but are not sure if the other person has similar feelings. They may be in a romantic relationship and wonder how the other person "truly" feels about them.

Whether directly or indirectly, friendships influence kids' and teens' health behaviors. Examples of friend influence include when, as too often occurs, the popular cliques exclude all but the "pretty people." Another example is the assumption in sports that an overweight person will not be as athletic, well-liked, or hardworking. That person may not be selected to play on a team or may be excluded from games. In and outside of school, these perceptions affect the way kids interact with their peers. A child may become apathetic because of being ignored.

In this chapter, you'll find strategies to discover what you need to know about your kids' friendships and how they fit into the health and wellness equation. Without snooping or being intrusive, you can open up a dialogue about friendships and how they are affecting your children's health behaviors. Relevant topics include whether they feel their friends are supportive of them when they are working toward goals, how their friends influence their health and weight management, and if they feel isolated as they are working through this. In addition, we'll look at other influences on kids' health behaviors, such as mass media and social media and the professionals with whom kids interact, such as teachers and coaches.

STRATEGY 37

ALL OF YOU

Examine Kids and Teens' Biological-Psychological-Social Makeup

You are witness to your kid or teen going through dramatic physical, cognitive, social, and emotional changes. To understand the factors that affect his health behaviors, all those changes need to be taken into consideration (referred to as "the Biopsychosocial Model").[105] To make real, fundamental change, the whole of your child needs to be paid attention to and supported.

From a biological perspective, your child is undergoing significant growth spurts as he advances through puberty. A majority of girls typically start their sexual development between ages eight and thirteen and have significant growth spurts from ten to fourteen. Most boys start developing sexually between the ages of ten to thirteen and continue growing until sixteen years of age.

Because of their hormonally driven changes, it is extremely important for tweens and teens to have well-balanced meals and to learn to eat healthily, engage in physical activity, and get adequate sleep. This ensures proper development and continued growth throughout this stage of life. Also, because of the rapid changes occurring in their bodies, understandably, many teens feel uncomfortable about their bodies for a while until they can adapt.

On a cognitive level, by his teen years your child understands responsibility and is able to reason and consider multiple viewpoints. He has the ability to integrate knowledge about healthful eating and exercising into his life and can problem solve challenging situations that could potentially stop him from engaging in healthful behaviors.

Psychologically, your child wants to win your approval by demonstrating specific competencies. If you encourage him, he'll receive positive

152

reinforcement for his initiatives, and he'll feel confident in his ability to set and achieve his health goals. If he is not encouraged, he can end up feeling inferior and doubting his own abilities.

As he further matures from childhood to adulthood, he seeks independence but also wants to fit in. He is figuring out what roles he will occupy as an adult and seeking to "find himself." If he fails to establish a sense of identity, he questions his place in society.[106] Lack of confidence, especially when comparing himself to others, may result in his feeling hopeless and inferior to his peers. When it comes to health goals, he may quickly give up (or not try at all) because of a belief that his efforts simply won't amount to anything.

His friends are the be all and end all. When you try to provide him with guidance, you may be rejected because you don't "get" him, and he most often "knows better" than you do. The difficulty is that he is at a stage where he wants more independence, but because of his teen ego, raging hormones, and at times impulsive behavior, he is actually in need of more support and supervision, not less.

During this stage, your child will also most likely have a sense of invincibility and immortality. He may think he doesn't have to take his health seriously and that he can wait to pay attention to it in the future when he is older.

According to a major study conducted by the Centers for Disease Control and Prevention, high school students are known to engage in unhealthy dietary behaviors such as not eating a nutritionally based diet with the recommended amount of fruits and vegetables, drinking sugared beverages, and not eating breakfast consistently. Also, they are not participating in enough physical activity during the week, are skipping out of physical education classes at school, are watching television for three or more hours a day, are on their computers for three or more hours a day, and are often not playing on at least one sports team run by their school or community group.

Additionally, nearly half (48 percent) are trying to lose weight, and 5 percent are resorting to using diet pills, laxatives, or vomiting to lose weight or to keep from gaining weight.[107] The sad fact is that only 10 percent will maintain their weight loss; the rest will be overweight or obese into adulthood. It is obvious that just working through this challenge on the physiological and nutritional level is not enough. *The psychological and social components are equally important to address this challenge, taking the whole kid or teen into account.* The following exercise will help you

153

consider all aspects of your child's development and how it affects his eating and exercise behaviors.

————

EXERCISE: Seeing Your Child Fully

Kids often feel that their parents don't "get" them. They resist parental help because they interpret it as criticism. In this exercise you'll write down where you think your child is from a developmental perspective, so that you can more easily see the whole child and be unconditionally supportive of him.

Physiological/biological makeup (e.g., large body frame, peanut allergy, etc.): _____
_____
_____

How might this affect healthful behaviors? _____
_____
_____
_____

Psychological makeup (e.g., anxiety, emotionally sensitive, etc.):
_____
_____
_____

How might this afffect healthful behaviors? _____
_____
_____
_____

Social makeup (e.g., introvert, mostly socializes with kids from camp rather than school, etc.): _____
_____
_____

How might this affect healthful behaviors? _____
_____
_____
_____

What health barriers might come up due to these factors?
_____

How do you feel when you think of the various elements you commented on? (For example, you feel frustrated because sociability doesn't come easily to your child.) _____

_____

_____

_____

How might you address them for yourself and for your child (what resources might be helpful, how might you choose to communicate about it to your child, etc.)? _____

_____

_____

_____

By assessing these factors, you can preemptively address challenges that may get in the way of your child's sticking to a healthful practice.

STRATEGY 38

GET PAST CULTURAL BIASES

Deal with Social and Marketing Influences

Being a modern-day kid comes with challenges. There are many pressures from outside sources that may sometimes take away from the joys of growing up. If your child is overweight or obese, she is likely struggling with additional pressures stemming from the media and our cultural obsession with thinness. In addition, there are intense pressures related to the constant bombardment of information on social media—Instagram, Snapchat, Facebook, and Twitter depict their peers and celebrities as having fun, being social, and looking perfect, and this can lead to unrealistic expectations. The biases in our society about being overweight or obese may lead your child to fear that she is not fitting into the "ideal," which may promote low self-confidence, isolation, and shame.

Your child is seeing images in the media for many hours each day. Some examples of how social media is affecting kids' self-perception and body image include their posting videos on YouTube of themselves asking, "Am I ugly?", posting selfies on Instagram with the hashtag #imugly,

#notugly, etc., or not receiving "likes" or instead receiving negative feedback. Whether eager for validation or posting in pride, they are leaving themselves vulnerable to criticism and cyberbullying by putting themselves out there in such an overt, public way.

Your child has most likely heard the sentiment that being overweight is unattractive. She may fear that if she becomes too overweight, she will not get married or ever have an intimate partner. She has also most likely heard that overweight people are not good athletes and are less likely to get picked for a team. These messages are often internalized because of what your child has heard, observed, or personally experienced.

Your child is also confronted with stereotypes that overweight people are lazy or unmotivated, have no discipline or willpower, are impulsive, like all things in excess, and are to blame for their circumstances. These biases are so embedded in our culture that we often do not realize when we are exposed to and affected by them.

TECHNOLOGY AND INSTANT GRATIFICATION

Your child lives in a fast-paced world where there is constant motion and stimulation from her TV, computer, smartphone, and other media—she probably rarely if ever unplugs. The pace of media reinforces her need for perpetual movement in order to pay attention and maintain focus. This high-speed input has a negative impact on her ability to tolerate delayed gratification and hinders your child from taking the necessary time to process, problem solve, and build up frustration tolerance. This also leads to unrealistic expectations, intense pressure, and exhaustion.

Many parents I spoke to while conducting my research expressed concern about their kids needing instant gratification and how they feel this carries over to their eating and exercise behaviors and their perception of themselves. One mother said, "When my son wants something to eat, it has to be now, at that moment, and not a moment later." Another mother said, "My daughter doesn't know how to be uncomfortable, not even for a minute. How is she ever going to withstand a craving or hold off from eating something she wants but that isn't the healthiest of choices?" This can also leave kids feeling frustrated when they don't see results or feel as if their hard work is going unnoticed.

If this describes your child, review Chapters 2 and 4 on mindfulness-based eating, and have your child take inventory of her hunger and cravings. Sitting with discomfort, working through cravings, and delaying

156

gratification are all skills that can help get kids connected to their hunger cues and more mindful of their eating. Additionally, remind them to use the six steps for taking ACTION, continually practice their skills, and make SMART goals (covered in Chapters 5 and 6) in order to see progress.

ADVERTISING AND MARKETING

More kids are overweight and obese today than ever before.[108] The media contributes to this epidemic by marketing unhealthful eating and drinking. Beverage companies spent $866 million to advertise such drinks as sodas and caffeinated energy drinks in 2013, four times as much as they spent advertising fruit juice and water. The number of ads for children's drinks on youth websites increased by 15 percent from 2010 to 2013.[109]

Despite promises by major companies to be part of the solution in addressing childhood obesity, reports show that companies continue to market their unhealthful products directly to children and teens. They have also rapidly expanded marketing in social and mobile media that are popular with young people and are much more difficult for parents to monitor.

PORTRAYAL OF THE "IDEAL"

While commercials coax kids into choosing unhealthy foods and beverages, your child is also exposed to the race for the skinny "ideal" and the undercurrent that thin is "better" and "more desirable" and leads to success and happiness. She sees this sentiment conveyed by the way magazines and other media portray the airbrushed waif models who are 5 feet 11 inches tall, weigh 117 pounds, and essentially make up 2 percent of the entire population. It is no wonder that 69 percent of girls in 5th through 12th grades reported that magazine pictures influenced their idea of a perfect body shape.[110]

This is also seen in the desire to fit into "skinny jeans" and striving for a thigh gap and protruding collarbone, which kids aspire to despite being unrealistic and unhealthy. There are numerous magazine articles and online instructional videos on how to achieve these ideals.

Given all that your child is experiencing and exposed to, it isn't surprising that she may be left with misperceptions and distorted views about her weight, body image, and health in general. It is important to take an inventory of what her perceptions are and to educate her about how they are being influenced and could perhaps change.

___

EXERCISE: Cultural Impact

Do this exercise with your child. Look at information being conveyed across all forms of media: social media, print media, TV, etc.

What are some examples of explicit and implicit messages communicating that "thin" is better and more favorable?

_____

_____

_____

_____

How often do you see examples of our weight-obsessed culture?

_____

_____

_____

_____

How often do you see examples of discrimination and biases against individuals who are overweight or obese?

_____

_____

_____

_____

FOOD AND BEVERAGE MARKETING

How often are foods and beverages that are low in nutrients advertised? How about advertisements specifically geared to kids and teens?

_____

_____

_____

_____

What terminology is used for foods indicating that they are being judged as bad or good? (e.g., "junk" food, "wrong" food, "bad" food, etc.) Where have you observed this?

_____

_____

_____

_____

Look at magazines (*Teen Vogue, Seventeen, Tiger Beat, Sports Illustrated*, etc.), TV, and online media and take notice of the models; what do you notice about their body proportions (height, weight, body structure, etc.)? Specifically, are the models representative of the average teen and advertising merchandise appropriate for teens? If not, why do you think they are not?

_____

_____

_____

_____

VERBAL FEEDBACK

What sentiments were communicated to you by family, friends, or anyone else regarding the consequences of being overweight (e.g., you won't be liked or get a boyfriend/girlfriend)?

_____

_____

_____

_____

IMPACT ON YOU

How did all of these influences shape how you think and feel about your weight? Your body? Your desire to lose weight? Other overweight or obese individuals?

_____

_____

_____

_____

How do you feel after doing this exploration? What did you learn that was most impactful?

_____

_____

_____

_____

STRATEGY 39

BULLYING IS NEVER OKAY

Work Through Bullying and Weight Discrimination

The prevalence of weight discrimination has significantly increased in recent decades and is comparable to the rates of racial discrimination.[111] Teasing about weight is more common than teasing about sexual orientation, race/ethnicity, physical disability, or religion.[112] Weight is the main reason for teasing and bullying at school.[113] There are multiple forms of weight bias, which include physical assault, verbal teasing (name-calling or derogatory remarks), and relational victimization (being ignored, excluded from activities, cyberbullied, and/or being the target of rumors).[114]

It's not only peers at school doing the teasing. Teachers may also have biases. Some teachers express that overweight students are untidy, more emotional, less likely to succeed at work, and more likely to have family problems.[115] They also have lower expectations for overweight students as compared to their thinner students.[116]

Kids who experience weight discrimination are more vulnerable to negative impacts on their physical, psychological, and social health. They are at significant risk for psychiatric disorders,[117] including depression, anxiety, low self-esteem, poor body image, and suicidal thoughts,[118] as well as disordered eating, avoidance of physical activity,[119] weight gain,[120] poor academic performance,[121] and social isolation.[122]

Weight bias exists because of the false beliefs that overweight and obese kids are to blame for their weight and could change their circumstances if they worked harder at it, that "tough love" and shaming will motivate them to embrace good health, and that thinness is more attractive and leads to greater success. There is a need for schools to offer community education to dispel these myths and direct interventions that assist kids who are being teased and bullied. Kids express a desire for

160

intervention and prefer to be supported by first their friends, followed by their peers, teachers, physical education (PE) teachers/coaches, and last, by their parents.[123]

There is little protection or recourse for kids who have experienced weight discrimination by way of teasing or bullying. State laws and local school policies address bullying but vary greatly across the country. There are no federal anti-bullying laws, and only three states include weight and appearance in their bullying policies: Maine, New Hampshire, and New York.[124] It is obvious that fundamental change needs to take place to adequately protect the plethora of kids who are being discriminated against.

A majority of parents of overweight children I interviewed reported that the schools their children attended intervened minimally, and if they did, it was done on the "micro level" (with their child), as opposed to the "macro level" (the entire school), including teacher training, anti-bullying education for students, etc. Also, parents reported that schools would intervene immediately only in circumstances where there was physical assault or threat of assault. Otherwise, the teasing or cyberbullying wasn't taken as seriously.

Many parents also reported to me that, in hindsight, if given the opportunity, they would have handled a bullying situation differently. They felt that they were reactive and responded too quickly and aggressively because of the rage and frustration evoked. Parents often over-identified with their children's plight, whether weight-related or otherwise. They also reported that they would now opt to listen more intently to how their children would prefer to handle the situation, rather than dictating how it "should" be handled.

It is not surprising that as a parent you would be compelled to come to your child's immediate aid because of an injustice he is experiencing. You would be prompted by your maternal/paternal instinct to protect him. Your discomfort is understandable. You are not expected to know how to intervene, as you were likely never taught how.

Your child's age, the severity of the discrimination, and his reaction to it will dictate how much to intervene. For example, for a younger or more immature child, you would intervene more extensively, because he may not be able to navigate the situation himself. At any age, if there is physical assault, or your child refuses or is fearful to attend school, you should intervene quickly and directly. These are general guidelines you can follow.

If your child confides in you that he is being teased or bullied at school (and there is no threat of physical assault):

1. Be ready to be fully present with your child. Focus on him, actively listen with intent and openness, and offer emotional support (for example, ask him what he needs in the moment), no matter what feelings are evoked in you. While addressing his needs, be aware of your feelings and make efforts to address them so that they won't impinge on the support you can offer him.

2. Avoid lecturing him, threatening to go to the school to confront the teasing child(ren), or immediately going to the teacher or administrator with this issue.

3. Actively and empathetically listen to any of the details of the teasing and/or bullying, even if minimal, that he is willing to offer you. He may not take advantage of your offer to have an open dialogue about it, particularly if he is feeling ashamed (that this is happening to him, that he cannot seem to effectively handle it himself, etc.), has the idea that you are disappointed in him (that he is overweight, which is causing this issue, that he cannot stick up for himself, etc.), or fears that you will not fully understand him (because you are not a kid, because you do not have this issue, etc.). Let him know that you are available at any time if and when he wants to share more.

4. Weight discrimination may specifically be covered under state anti-bullying laws and school anti-bullying policies. They vary considerably from state to state and school to school. Find out what your school's policies are around teasing and bullying and whether they have a protocol in place to handle these situations. You may elect to confidentially speak to a school social worker or psychologist, if there is one available, or a trusted member of the administration for guidance.

5. Ask your child what he wants and what he thinks his options are. Fill in the blanks for him if he does not raise options that are potentially viable. Narrow down the options and, together, identify the advantages and disadvantages of each. You can use pen and paper to chart this out.

ADVANTAGES OF APPROACHING THE TEACHER	DISADVANTAGES OF APPROACHING THE TEACHER
ADVANTAGES OF NOT APPROACHING THE TEACHER	DISADVANTAGES OF NOT APPROACHING THE TEACHER

6. After you and your child have completed the table with the advantages and disadvantages for each quadrant, ask your child to rank on a scale from 1 to 5 what each item's level of importance is to him (5 being most important and 1 being the least important). For example, an advantage of approaching the teacher is that the teacher can discuss the issue of teasing with the entire class without identifying your child as the person having the issue.

7. When you ask your child how important each item is to him, he may say a 4 for approaching the teacher and having a group discussion because another kid in the class is also being teased, and it might help him and others, as well. Another child may evaluate the same item as a 1 because he may have the perception that others in the class will figure out that it's him that the teacher is talking about.

8. Add up the numbers on the diagonal quadrants (advantages of approaching the teacher and disadvantages of not approaching the teacher, versus advantages of not approaching the teacher and disadvantages of approaching the teacher). Compare the two sets of numbers and discuss which is greater. If the numbers are close, discuss the conflict that is presenting itself.

9. Finalize a course of action once you find out what the school policies and protocol are and you have fully processed the options with your child.

On a macro level, administrators, teachers, and coaches should receive training about the biological, psychological, and social development of

163

the kids they work with. They also should be trained on the prevention and warning signs of obesity and eating disorders. Finally, they should be educated on the prevalence of weight bias and discrimination, how to address it, and awareness of their own biases (we all have them!) and how they affect their work with kids. You could personally choose to advocate for such training and model empowerment, advocacy, and assertiveness to your child.

STRATEGY 40

YOUR BODY IS AN EXTENSION OF YOU

Combating Self-Criticism

Our bodies are extensions of ourselves. If your child disdains parts of her body, it affects how she sees herself and could affect how she interacts with the world around her.

There is a distinction between the observing mind and the thinking mind.[125] With an observing mind, we are able to see ourselves just as we are, without adding judgments and criticisms. The thinking mind tends to get flooded with judgments and criticisms rather than simply seeing what is. These "add-ons" often have an impact on how we perceive ourselves and behave.

EXERCISE: Observing Yourself Neutrally

It is critical that your child become aware of how she views herself and her body. Awareness is key. When she has those inevitable self-critical thoughts (and we all have them sometimes), she can point it out to herself, recognize what is influencing them, and challenge her thinking to look at things in a new way. Whether with you or alone, have your child look in a full-length mirror. Have her take notice of her various body parts and write down the *first* thoughts that come to mind.

Face: _____

Hair: _____

Arms: _____

Hands: _____

Chest: _____

Thighs: _____

Legs: _____

Feet: _____

After completing this list, explain the difference between making an *observation* and making a *judgment*. For example, "I have a pimple on my face" is an observation. "I look like a nasty freak" is a judgment. Make it a point to highlight that we most often make negative *judgments* rather than neutral *observations* about ourselves and that, in doing so, we perpetuate negative thoughts and feelings. This cycle erodes self-confidence, self-acceptance, self-compassion, and self-love.

Following this, ask her to *observe herself just as she is without attaching anything to the observations*. For example, "My thighs are muscular, my nose is long, and I have a pimple on my face." Process this exercise with her. What thoughts and feelings come up for her as she just observes? For a day, encourage her to journal how often she makes negative self-judgments, how automatic that thinking is for her, and how it affects her feelings and behavior.

Ask your child to think about (and discuss, if she is open to it):

- How often do self-judgments come up?
- Are the judgments based on what the "ideals" are in society?
- Is there is a specific body part that you tend to fixate on?
- Are there parts that you think more negatively about than other parts?
- Are there parts that you may have a love/hate relationship with? How?
- Is there a part you would like to change? Why?
- What would you change it to look like?
- Why do you think it would look better that way?
- Are there body parts that you appreciate?
- Why do you appreciate them?

Stress the importance of noticing when the judgments come up for her and how she can reframe them. For example, how else can she see the situation with her pimple? She can acknowledge that she would prefer not to have the pimple and that it is making her uncomfortable. She could *also* notice that it's a pimple that is temporarily on her face and will eventually go away, that just because she has a pimple does not mean she is a freak, and that she ordinarily does not feel this way when the pimple is not there. A pimple does not define who she is.

To encourage gratitude toward her body and all it does to help her function, end the exercise by asking her to be thankful for and give loving kindness toward the body parts she described earlier. Have her go through each one: face, hair, arms, etc. For example, "I'm thankful for my face because it houses body parts that allow me to use my senses, such as sight, smell, hearing, and taste." Last, if she is willing, ask her to "give up" one of those parts for an hour to experiment with how it would feel not to have it. For example, bind her fingers together with a string, leaving her thumb out on her dominant hand, and have her go about her general functioning (e.g., doing homework, eating dinner, etc.). Process the experience with her afterward. This exercise helps her show compassion for herself while having gratitude for all parts of her, which are all equally important.

🧳 CHECK YOUR BAGGAGE

Think back—you remember what it was like to be a kid or teen, don't you? Most parents comment that they would never want to return to that time because it was so trying and confusing. And today's world is even more complicated than the one you grew up in. It is so complex, you wonder how your child is getting through it and worry all the time. How can you know how to help your child navigate health issues on top of all the challenges of adolescence or teenhood?

It's critical that you recognize that every child is unique and has a unique set of challenges. Be sure to try to understand your child fully, including their physiology and where they are emotionally and socially. Take note of any negative judgments you may feel, and make it a point to explore how you will lend support to them. Your child needs you fully and unconditionally.

You are obviously looking out for your child's best interests and want them to be unscathed by the cruelty of this world. If teasing or bullying has happened, be open to getting your own support to help them effectively work through this challenge. Your child is already having feelings about the circumstances; they need a supportive parent who can empathize and act as a guide.

You, too, are influenced by society's messages about ideals—we are all in the same boat. We all sometimes make negative judgments about our bodies and physical appearance—note what yours are, and be sure to model the behavior you are asking of your child.

Aim for an open dialogue with your child. Keep in mind that they may not agree with or buy into everything you convey, and that's okay. When your child has those reactions, be open, patient, understanding, and empathetic. Rather than cutting off these feelings prematurely, allow them to express themselves to you and talk with you about troubling thoughts and feelings. Be open to whatever comes up.

 ## REVIEW

You've gained an understanding about how your child is developing, the cultural ideals currently making an impact, how your child can be discriminated against because of weight, and how to handle self-criticism. Dealing with these factors appropriately can increase your child's self-confidence, self-acceptance, and self-love and is critical to healthful behaviors.

Parents can:

- Understand the whole child—from a biological, psychological, and social framework—and recognize their unique challenges, and empower their strengths.
- Talk about how cultural ideals influence how both of you view and experience your general weight and health.
- Understand the ramifications of teasing and bullying, and take steps to effectively deal with them.
- Gain insight into your child's disparaging self-criticisms—are they negatively judging instead of simply observing?—and help reframe this thinking.
- Help your child have focused awareness and gratitude for their body.

 ## MINDFULNESS EXERCISE: Awareness of Your Body

See page 225 for the mindfulness exercise that corresponds to this chapter, and refer to page 217 for instructions on accessing the audio.

9

Active Living

> I don't like exercising. I don't know why people say that it makes them feel better. When I tried, it just made me feel achy and exhausted. I'm not going to do something that makes me feel that way.
>
> —FIONA, AGE 15

> Who has time for exercising? I have to worry about college applications, studying for the SATs, homework, and getting together with friends. I can't fit it in. —DYLAN, AGE 17

ALTHOUGH TEENS SOMETIMES SEE exercise as a chore, there is no reason it has to be experienced that way. There truly is an enjoyable physical activity for everyone. Done consistently, exercise will fortify your child's confidence, personal strength, and overall commitment to self-love and self-care.

In this chapter, you and your child will learn why exercising is beneficial, how much exercise your child needs for a healthy lifestyle, what types of activities can be actively engaged in, and what sabotages exercising efforts. Throughout, there are examples of how kids can respond to unhelpful thoughts and feelings about exercising, as well as realistic recommendations for integrating physical activity into their lives.

This chapter highlights what may be getting in the way of your child adopting a more physically active lifestyle. Often, feelings of frustration about exercise end up preventing your child from sustaining the motivation to act. Other factors that affect your child's participation may include how physical education and sports are structured in and out of school, the weather and the opportunity to play outdoors, the neighborhood you live in, and the affordability of activities.

You'll learn how to help your kids set realistic goals and how to make exercise an ongoing practice. This includes tips on time management, setting up personal goals and challenges, and securing support to create a sustainable practice. It's also important to teach kids and teens about getting in touch with the way the body functions, a skill that's important for lifelong weight maintenance and general well-being.

We'll also talk about ways to make exercise social and fun. While it's true that your child may not be enthusiastic to outright exercise with you, you can still find ways to be active as a family and organize groups of friends who get outdoors in a fun, informal way.

Finally, you will be able to help your child respond to rationalizations and unhelpful thoughts regarding exercising. You can help your child write power cards (see page 182) to be fully prepared when these thoughts arise and to mindfully and effectively deal with them. Parents can also go through the process of journaling with their children (see page 56) so that the whole family can commit to actively participating in healthful practices.

STRATEGY 41

THE POWER OF MOVEMENT

Take Advantage of the Benefits of Exercise

Exercise is a key factor leading to the long-term maintenance of weight and health management. Studies consistently find that people who exercise the most also have the most weight loss and improved health.[126] Exercise has numerous benefits and greatly contributes to a mindful approach to health. Explain these important benefits to your child:

- **EXERCISE BOOSTS ACADEMIC PERFORMANCE:** In one study, girls who exercised regularly demonstrated a significant improvement in science performance, and at ages fifteen and sixteen, every additional seventeen minutes of exercise a day for boys and twelve minutes for girls was linked to better examination results.[127] In other studies, exercise significantly affected memory, learning,[128] and cognition.[129]
- **EXERCISE CONTROLS WEIGHT:** It can prevent excess weight gain and help maintain healthy weight. We burn calories during exercise. Depending on the intensity, you can burn fewer or more calories during any physical activity.

- **EXERCISE BOOSTS ENERGY:** It improves muscle strength and boosts endurance. It delivers oxygen and nutrients to your tissues so that the cardiovascular system works more efficiently. When your major organs work more efficiently, you have more energy overall.

- **EXERCISE COMBATS DISEASE:** It strengthens your heart and lungs. It can help prevent heart disease, stroke, type 2 diabetes, depression, osteoporosis, and arthritis, lower blood pressure, reduce the incidence of colon and breast cancers, boost high-density lipoproteins (HDL) or "good cholesterol," and decrease low-density lipoproteins (LDL) or "bad cholesterol."

- **EXERCISE HAS PSYCHOLOGICAL BENEFITS:** Besides improving mood, decreasing anxiety,[130] and increasing self-confidence, exercise stimulates brain chemicals called endorphins and neurotransmitters called serotonin that leave you feeling more positive and energetic. It also reduces perception of pain (what's personally challenging and emotionally uncomfortable), which directly improves mood.[131] It positively affects body image, the belief in one's ability to successfully complete tasks and accomplish goals (self-efficacy), and coping skills.[132]

- **EXERCISE JUMP-STARTS THE IMMUNE SYSTEM:** It helps reduce the number of colds, flu, and viruses you get.

- **EXERCISE KEEPS MUSCLES, JOINTS, AND BONES STRONG:** Strong muscles burn more calories because they are metabolically active tissue. The more muscle mass you have, the more calories you'll burn, even when you're not working out. Research shows that doing muscle-strengthening and bone-strengthening physical activity can slow the loss of bone density that naturally comes with age.[133] It also helps with agility, reflex/flexibility, and coordination in general and during sports performance.

- **EXERCISE PROMOTES BETTER SLEEP:** It can help you fall asleep faster and deepen your sleep.

- **EXERCISE EXTENDS LIFE:** According to the Centers for Disease Control and Prevention, people who are physically active for about seven hours a week have a 40 percent lower risk of dying early than those who are active for less than thirty minutes a week.[134]

170

EXERCISE: Return to Values

Your child is more likely to take on exercise as an ongoing practice if there is something personally meaningful that is driving her participation. Return to your child's values and what is meaningful to her (see Chapter 2). Ask her which benefits she connects to that represent why she would want to invest in exercise. She may feel passionate about playing sports and want to work on her performance by becoming better coordinated and more flexible (her value is sports/athleticism), or she may feel invested in her academic performance and want to improve her learning and memory (her value is learning/education).

She will also gain awareness about what direction she wants to take that is in line with her values and specifically what goals she needs to meet to effectively carry out those values.

HOW MUCH EXERCISE KIDS NEED—VERSUS HOW MUCH THEY ARE ACTUALLY GETTING

According to the CDC and the US Department of Health and Human Services, children ages six to seventeen should do an hour or more of physical activity each day.[135] Aerobic activity should make up most of this time. It can include a moderate or vigorous activity (at least three times a week), a muscle-strengthening activity such as gymnastics or push-ups (three times a week) and a bone-strengthening activity such as jumping rope or running (three times a week).

For example, a teen's daily exercise regimen may include: a one-mile walk on a treadmill before school; a one-mile walk around the track during school lunch period; a one-mile walk after school with friends or the dog; sports team practice (basketball, soccer, hockey, etc.).

Even though the CDC and US Department of Health have given their recommendations, kids and teens are still not getting nearly the amount of physical activity that they need. In 2013, only 17.7 percent of female high school students and 36.6 percent of male students were participating in at least sixty minutes of physical activity a day. Only 24 percent of females and 34.9 percent of males were attending physical education classes daily.[136]

In 2014, the National Physical Activity Plan Alliance wrote a comprehensive document using the report card system to evaluate physical activity for children and youth in the United States.[137] Here's what they looked at and how they graded kids' activity levels:

171

Overall physical activity (grade: D-)

Sedentary behaviors (grade: D)

Active transportation, such as walking or biking to school (grade: F)

Organized sports participation (grade: C-)

Active play (grade: incomplete [INC])

Health-related fitness (grade: INC)

Physical activity with family and peers (grade: INC)

Physical activity at school (grade: C-)

Physical activity in the community and built environment (grade: B-)

Government strategies and investments to promote children's physical activity (grade: INC)

These low grades show how many health resources your child is not currently receiving adequately or, for that matter, receiving at all. Now more than ever, parents must take initiative to ensure that their children are sufficiently participating in physical activity.

STRATEGY 42

MAKING THE TEAM

Identify Barriers to Exercise

Even if your child desires more physical activity, there may be factors that get in the way of his involvement. Identifying these barriers with your child is critical, as often misperceptions lead to inactivity. He may perceive himself as "lazy," "unwilling," or "not athletic." These thoughts are real to him and could strongly influence why he isn't participating. Understanding and dismantling these barriers can make exercise more accessible.

There are many influences on a child's participation: biological and demographic, psychological and social, and physical environment.[138] Males tend to exercise more than females, and if parents live an active lifestyle, their children are more likely to.[139] Your child also needs to believe that time can be found to exercise and that the personal benefits outweigh the costs. One of strongest predictors of success is confidence in one's ability to be active on a regular basis. And children especially are more likely to participate and continue participating if they enjoy what they are doing.[140]

Strenuous exertion was another deterrent for children.[141] They prefer activities with lower levels of exertion, and dropout rates are higher from vigorous activity than from moderate-intensity activities.[142] Other determinants include whether friends and family are role models, encourage physical activity, actively participate with their children, and directly help them to be physically active.[143]

In my focus groups, parents reported three more things as being major deterrents for their children when it came to physical activity. They shared that if their children felt shame or insecurity about their appearance, they were less likely to participate, that there wasn't a place for them to engage in physical activity if they were mediocre at sports, and that physical education isn't offered enough at school.

Parents unanimously reported that when they attended middle and high school, they engaged in more physical activity than their children currently do. Also, by the time their children came home from school, had a bit of downtime, and finished their homework, they were exhausted and didn't have enough time to fit anything else in.

APPEARANCE AND INSECURITY

Kids and teens are often confronted by situations that provoke shame regarding their weight and body size. In the focus groups I conducted, overweight teens (and many who were average weight, too) reported feeling most humiliated at school when they were forced to take fitness tests, as well as on an ongoing basis when they changed for gym class because of the expectation that they dress in shorts and tank tops. This made them feel insecure and embarrassed, and they found themselves comparing themselves to other students whom they perceived as thinner, more attractive, or more fit. All of these factors deterred them from wanting to participate.

COMPETITIVE SPORTS

Why do some kids stop exercising or never even start? Today's kids are 15 percent less aerobically fit than their parents were at their age.[144]

Competitive sports are one of the factors contributing to this statistic. When I was in high school, people could still make a varsity team if they were willing to put in the time and effort. Now, that's rarely the case, as so many kids begin competitive training as early as preschool and continue with that level of intensity well into elementary, middle, and high school.

For everyone else, it's often not enough anymore to just have fun playing a sport; most athletics for kids are organized and competitive. So where does that leave the rest of the kids and teens who are not skilled athletes? Or who like a sport but who may never be good enough to make the team? Or who don't even bother trying because they're anxious or intimidated from the outset? It's unfortunate that our kids are being socialized to believe that sports are more about competition than for having fun and engaging in a physical activity that promotes good health.

In activities such as tennis, gymnastics, swim, dance, etc., kids often start when they are in preschool or grammar school and advance as they get older. If a child discovers an interest in a sport in adolescence, it may require him to take classes or lessons with children much younger than he is. For example, at thirteen, my son decided to transition from skiing to snowboarding. His choices narrowed to taking lessons with adults who were beginners or had never skied, paying for expensive private lessons, or joining a group of seven- and eight-year-olds who were beginners, which he opted to do. If it weren't for his eight-year-old brother taking lessons at the time, he would have opted out and stayed with skiing, thereby missing out on learning a new sport that he was interested in.

PHYSICAL EDUCATION IN SCHOOLS

After analyzing kids' fitness for forty-six years, researchers have found that children's cardio endurance has decreased by 5 percent every decade.[145] If this trend continues, future generations are at grave risk of being more overweight and having more cardiovascular-related diseases. Because kids and teens spend most of their waking hours at school, it's a natural place where they should be engaging in physical activity.

There is no federal law that mandates physical education be provided in American schools. Individual states establish guidelines, but there is no uniformity in regard to the amount of PE required, class size, whether there are exceptions made, whether they follow a state curriculum, whether a fitness assessment is required, how fitness is assessed, whether the grade is included in the student's grade point average (GPA), whether body mass index (BMI) is calculated, whether PE teachers need a certification or license, and whether they have a district PE coordinator. All of these factors vary from state to state.[146] There are also no state PE requirements for private schools. The lack of firm requirements reduces the likelihood that schools will adhere to the state guidelines.[147]

My research exposed glaring issues that came up regarding certain requirements that have an impact on kids' and teens' physical activity participation. The state of New York, where I conducted my research, requires a student assessment in PE in grades 1 through 12. This assessment typically includes flexibility, upper body muscle strength and endurance, abdominal muscle strength and endurance, aerobic endurance, and body composition.

For many overweight kids and teens I spoke to, this process is extremely anxiety-inducing. They felt anxiety anticipating the assessment and shame and humiliation during the process and often reported experiencing name-calling or bullying by their peers during and after the assessment. Another reported issue was how PE instructors conveyed feedback to students about their assessment results and BMI; it was gingerly recommended that students participate more often in physical activity. When I asked if that was helpful in any way, unanimously these students reported that it wasn't, because they didn't have any support for following through with the recommendations, and they didn't feel that there was a place for them to participate that would meet their fitness levels.

The recommendation by the National Association of Sports and Physical Education (NASPE) and the American Heart Association is that elementary students be offered 150 minutes a week of physical education and middle and high school students 225 minutes per week throughout the school year. There's good reason for these recommendations—the obvious benefits of exercise on focusing and learning. In some cases, inactivity in school and difficulty with sitting still can also lead to improper diagnosis of attention deficit hyperactivity disorder (ADHD).[148]

Even with the evident benefits, only six states nationwide require the recommended 150 minutes of elementary school–based PE. In forty-one states, middle school PE is mandated, and in forty-four states, high school PE is mandated.[149] In New York, where I reside, for grades 7–12, the regulations require PE three times per week in one semester and twice per week in the second.[150] Each period extends on the average for forty to forty-five minutes. Assuming the schools are adhering to the requirements, teens are only getting on the average 80 to 135 minutes of

PE per week. This number is exceedingly lower than the national recommendations. And yet high school is a time when the need for exercise is even more critical—because of teens' level of stress due to preparation for college, where they are developmentally due to hormonal changes, and because the practice sets them up for healthy habits into adulthood.

For many years, schools have reduced or eliminated PE and sports programming, given budget cuts and the greater emphasis on academic performance. When conducting my research, I spoke to PE directors in the state of New York about the inadequate amount of time high school students in particular are getting for PE. I was frequently told that there isn't enough time because of academics and that there are athletic offerings at school (junior varsity, varsity, modified, intramurals, clubs, open gyms, etc.) that students can join to supplement their physical activity hours at school. They agreed that the students who need the physical activity the most are the unlikeliest ones to join the teams or take advantage of the resources because of feeling ashamed, intimidated, or not physically fit enough, or due to physical disabilities and/or limitations, and expressed that it is an ongoing and enduring issue.

PHYSICAL ENVIRONMENT AND SOCIAL DETERMINANTS

A child's environment also affects participation in physical activity—everything from the weather, safety outdoors near the home, to whether there are adequate resources in the neighborhood (parks, facilities, programs that are convenient and affordable, etc.).[151] Social determinants are another factor: whether friends and family are role models, encourage physical activity, and actively participate and directly help kids and teens to be physically active.

Now that you have a sense of the many factors related to your child's physical activity, you can assess his level of participation in general and what might be getting in the way. Then, you can work toward providing resources for him so he can increase his activity.

EXERCISE: Assess Your Child's Participation

Have your child assess his level of physical activity over a two-week period.

How much cardiovascular activity are you getting on a daily basis?

(Distinguish between in-school and out-of-school hours.)

Monday _____ Tuesday _____ Wednesday _____

Thursday _____ Friday _____ Saturday _____ Sunday _____

TOTAL # OF HOURS _____

How much strength training activity are you getting on a daily basis? (Distinguish between in-school and out-of-school hours.)

Monday _____ Tuesday _____ Wednesday _____

Thursday _____ Friday _____ Saturday _____ Sunday _____

TOTAL # OF HOURS _____
TOTAL HOURS PER WEEK: Week 1 _____ Week 2 _____

How close is it to the 60 minutes a day that is recommended by the CDC? _____

In school, how close is it to the 150 minutes (middle school) or 225 minutes (high school) per week that is recommended? _____

What is keeping you from engaging in PE at school? (*Check all those that apply*)

- ❏ They don't offer it enough at school.
- ❏ There is a lack of programming for my fitness level.
- ❏ I can't make it on a team.
- ❏ I feel embarrassed or intimidated.
- ❏ Other _____

These are the ten most common reasons people don't adopt a more physically active lifestyle.[152] Which ones apply to you?

- ❏ Don't have enough time
- ❏ Find it inconvenient
- ❏ Lack self-motivation
- ❏ Do not find exercise enjoyable
- ❏ Find it boring
- ❏ Lack confidence in my ability to be physically active
- ❏ Fear being injured or have been injured recently
- ❏ Lack self-management skills, such as the ability to set personal goals, monitor progress, or reward progress toward such goals

❏ Lack support, encouragement, or companionship from family and friends

❏ Do not have parks, sidewalks, bicycle trails, or safe and pleasant walking paths convenient to my home

❏ Other_____

❏ Other_____

In order to understand what mechanisms to put in place to help your child participate in physical activity, it is important to get a sense of the barriers that get in his way. Some barriers may be external and can be problem solved (see Chapter 5 on problem-solving skills to work through this), while others are internal and could be due to his thinking. His mind may attempt to convince him that he can't do it, and if he takes that as a fact, he won't. Next, we'll look at thoughts that can sabotage his efforts and how to get past them.

STRATEGY 43

GET IN ON THE ACTION

Try These Fitness Tips

As a parent, you have limited control over the structure and culture of athletics today and what happens at school. But you can be proactive in other arenas. Here are tips that you can share with your child to boost her confidence and help facilitate her exercising. Ask your child, "Which tips speak to you? Which ones can you relate to? Which do you predict may be more challenging than others on this list? How will you get through these challenges?"

- Schedule exercise as you would any appointment. To help with time management, set aside specific days and times for exercising, and reschedule for the same week as needed.
- Start slowly and gradually increase your level of activity over time. If you start too quickly, you may burn out before reaping the rewards of your efforts. That means you could become frustrated because your muscles are sore, feel disappointed for being unable to accomplish what you thought you could, or experience exhaustion from pushing yourself too hard.
- You also don't have to exercise all at one time. You can break it

up throughout the day. You should find what works for you.

- We inevitably have unhelpful thoughts that help us rationalize why we don't have to be exercising. We can have the thought and still exercise. Remember, Mind over Muffin! (See page 26.)

- Most people claim they really tried and give up before they can see results. For them, trying is usually defined as a week or two of consistent exercising. It takes a lot longer to really notice a change. We stick it out a lot longer for other things when we're waiting for change to occur. For example, you would tolerate wearing braces so that your teeth are straightened. Healing from a broken leg takes weeks, and you would wait that time out. Real change takes time, patience, and genuine effort.

- Go with your gut and be keenly aware of how your body feels while you're exercising. If something hurts and is uncomfortable, vary what you're doing and assert yourself if you're exercising with someone. No one knows your body as well as you do!

- Accept that this may not come easily for you and that you may need to motivate yourself to stay on track. Identify specific motivators, such as having a healthy lunch afterward or reading a book that you intended to read, to help keep you committed.

- Nike got it right with its slogan: "Just do it." You don't have to start out motivated in order to exercise! Action often initiates motivation rather than the other way around. Once you feel more accomplished, more energetic, and physically better, you are more likely to continue exercising. Most people are not raring to go from the beginning, so you're not alone.

- Exercise is as necessary for us as a walk is to a dog. If you're thinking of giving up, ask whether you would think that about taking your dog for a walk. Would you say, "He needs it and it's good for him, but I won't do it because it's doing the same thing every day, and I don't feel like it"? Hopefully not!

- Your body is an extension of you. Each body part and its functions are equally important. If your leg was broken, would you neglect going to a doctor? Why is it okay to neglect vital organs such as the heart and lungs?

- Everything you want to get positive results from takes continuous, conscious effort. Just as schoolwork and even brushing your teeth takes effort, so does maintaining physical fitness.

- You won't ever *have* the time—you need to *make* the time for exercising.
- Any amount of exercise is helpful, even if it isn't as much as you intended. Any exercise is better than no exercise.
- Anyone can exercise when they feel like it. But doing it when you are not in the mood is even more important to boost mood and self-confidence.
- Before you exercise, remind yourself of the positive benefits (e.g., improved mood, better sleep, more energy, and better academic performance) and the fact that you will almost invariably feel better afterward.
- Praise and acknowledge yourself after exercise. You're doing something meaningful for your health. You deserve appreciation for your efforts.
- Integrate exercise into family time. This will provide you with a method to bond with family members, relieve stress, and maintain a healthy lifestyle. You and your family members will learn invaluable lifelong skills for staying fit and healthy and will enjoy doing so in the process. Activities can include hiking, skiing, roller-blading, ice skating, speed walking, biking, etc.
- Building confidence is what will propel you to move forward and maintain your practice. The best way to do this is to actually exercise and prove to yourself that you are capable.

These tips can help your child get in on the action and participate in physical activity. Additionally, these are ways that you can be directly involved in helping your child. When you exercise yourself, you will be positively modeling the skills that you want your child to learn, and your child will feel more supported in her efforts.

Physical activity that's personally chosen based on your child's preference and ability can be a great source of fitness and pleasure. Be mindful in regard to the way you communicate about exercising, because it can directly affect her willingness to participate. Avoid sending the message that participating in exercise and fitness is a punishment for eating the wrong foods ("I have to exercise twice as hard tomorrow because I ate that bread") or that the main reason to participate is to change her body ("I need to workout to get rid of my flabby abs"). Foster sentiments that convey that exercise is fun and makes us feel good.[153]

OVERCOME "I CAN'T, I WON'T"

Power Cards for Fitness

There are many barriers that may get in the way of you and your child actively participating in exercise and fitness. We all know exercise is beneficial, but even for adults, there are barriers to getting to the gym or going outside for a hike. Our thoughts have a way of convincing us that we are not ready or able, don't have enough time, or won't ever succeed. In order to maintain an exercise regimen, your child needs to respond to those unhelpful thoughts and work toward living his values.

The reassuring fact is that he gets to choose how he exercises and how often. It's okay for him to be selective and find what works for him. He is more likely to stick with it if he enjoys what he's choosing to do.

EXERCISE: Identify Negative Thoughts

Ask your child to use the following list to check off the unhelpful thoughts that hold him back from exercising. (*Check all those that apply*)

- ❏ I'm not an exercise person.
- ❏ I don't like to sweat.
- ❏ I get out of breath too quickly.
- ❏ I'm much more of a _____ kid and not an athlete.
- ❏ I'm not good at it.
- ❏ I don't know how to exercise.
- ❏ I don't like being sore.
- ❏ I don't like the way I look when I exercise.
- ❏ I don't like to do it alone.
- ❏ I don't have anywhere to exercise.
- ❏ Why start? I'm never going to be able to keep this up.
- ❏ I have too much school work.
- ❏ Other _____

EXERCISE: Create Power Cards for Exercising

Have your child create his own power cards based on the items he checked off as thoughts that get in the way of exercising. He can fill out as many as he wants to. He can also laminate them and carry them with him to assist with rationalizations and unhelpful thoughts.

POWER CARD

UNHELPFUL THOUGHT:

I don't have the time to exercise.

HELPFUL REPLIES:

1. I will never have the time—I need to make the time.

2. I need to make this a priority, or else I will not meet the goals I set out to achieve.

3. I don't have to earmark extensive time periods; I can exercise at 15- or 30-minute intervals.

4. I can add physical activity to my daily routine— walking the dog, biking, walking to school, using the stairs instead of the elevator, etc.

5. I could ask family and friends to participate.

6. I can make it part of my weekly schedule and write it in my calendar or planner.

POWER CARD

UNHELPFUL THOUGHT:

I don't know how to exercise. I'm afraid I'll injure myself.

HELPFUL REPLIES:

1. I'm not expected to know how to exercise, but I can learn.

2. Just because I don't know how to do something doesn't mean I should give up on it. I didn't know how to drive before I learned how to—imagine if I had given up on that.

3. I'm going to commit to learning how to warm up and cool down to prevent injury.

4. I'm going to choose activities that have minimal risk.

5. The more fit I am, the less likely I am to injure myself.

By making and using power cards, your child can establish what rationalizations tend to come up, reframe the way he thinks about them, and impose more mindful, balanced thinking, which will ultimately affect his behavior.

STRATEGY 45

ACTIVELY ENGAGE

Get Involved and Track Participation

Getting involved with your child's exercise participation is key. Most kids and teens want their parents to be actively involved and provide direct support. What does that mean? Here are some ways parents can help:

- Have equipment on hand that encourages physical activity (basketball hoop, soccer and hockey net, etc.).
- Go to places that foster physical activity (parks, baseball fields, basketball courts, etc.).
- Remain positive about and active in children's sports activities.
- Encourage your child while she is participating, and drive her to and from activities if she isn't driving yet.
- Be respectful of who your child is and whether she prefers group or solo activities. As long as she participates, it doesn't matter what her preference is.
- Show your child a variety of activities and enable her to choose what she enjoys doing. Make activities fun whether they are structured or unstructured. It could be doing a program on the elliptical machine or taking a hike in the woods near your home.
- Limit screen time (the recommendation is no more than two hours a day), and, whenever possible, encourage your child to play outdoors.
- If physical-activity resources aren't readily available in your neighborhood, drive, bike, or walk to gain access.
- If resources aren't easily accessible or available at all or your child prefers to exercise in private or individually, use cost-effective or no-cost alternative methods that can be accessed at home, such as streaming videos, fitness apps, DVDs, etc. (See Resources for a list.)
- Reorganize your child's schedule to include time for exercising. She may need to give something up or adjust her schedule.
- Identify what your child needs in order to remain organized and scheduled. There is greater chance for success when exercise is part of her routine and she knows that.
- Encourage your child to set SMART goals while exercising (see Chapter 6 for a refresher on SMART goals). This helps to diminish boredom so your child remains interested, challenged, and invested.
- Identify some forms of physical activity that appeal to your child. It should ideally be low to moderate intensity, not take a lot of time, and be convenient, relatively painless, and possibly fun or social. If your child feels embarrassed doing it, it is not for her. She will be less likely to stick to it in the long run.
- If your child is not interested in team sports, encourage her to

select more individualized, less competitive, or noncompetitive activities, such as horseback riding, jumping rope, catching and throwing a ball, shooting baskets, riding a bike, etc.

- When your child starts exercising, and if it's financially feasible, consider hiring a personal trainer so your child can learn proper form, alignment, and exercise safety. You can arrange for this at home, at a gym (usually restricted to teens sixteen and older), or at a private studio. You could check local listings in your area or ask for a referral.
- Keep a range of activities in mind so your child has options for the amount of time she has, the weather, availability of friends, etc.
- Encourage your child to participate in physical activity, but don't force her to participate.
- Always take into consideration how convenient it will be to perform the activity and how much time it will take.

EXERCISE: Create a Daily Log

Your child should fill out this daily log for a week and earmark specific times during those days for exercise, as well as types of activities that she'll commit to performing.

DAY OF WEEK	CARDIOVASCULAR ACTIVITIES	MUSCLE-STRENGTHENING ACTIVITIES
MONDAY		
TUESDAY		
WEDNESDAY		
THURSDAY		
FRIDAY		
SATURDAY		
SUNDAY		

After you have reviewed the barriers, provided tips, and facilitated the support to make it possible for your child to participate, she will be ready to set up a schedule and create her goals for exercising. You are actively helping your child make positive changes and improve her health, and she will greatly benefit from your attention, support, and care.

CHECK YOUR BAGGAGE

We all have extremely busy and full schedules, and sometimes the idea of adding anything more to yours or your child's schedule can be over-whelming. Personal feelings may come up about the amount of exercise that is recommended and your ability to help your child carry it out. It's important to get in touch with feelings and thoughts that may get in the way of supporting your child through this process.

If you face this task with resistance, hesitation, or dismay, your child may pick up on your feelings and be less open to integrating fitness goals for improved health. As noted, there are external barriers to exercise that you and your child may have little control over. You can be proactive by advocating on behalf of your child and securing resources so that your child has a greater chance of integrating exercise into a daily schedule and sustaining it as an ongoing practice.

There are sabotaging thoughts that may show up for your child that are a deterrent to exercising. You may be able to relate to these thoughts or feel frustration that they show up. Be aware of your thoughts and feelings so that they don't negatively affect your ability to provide the support that your child may need from you.

Be aware of the ways you can get directly involved with your child's exercise practice. If you personally need extra support to effectively help, take the initiative so both of you can benefit. Participating in activities as a family can be encouraging and connecting. There are great benefits when, collectively, family members feel challenged, strengthened, and empowered.

REVIEW

Invest in exercising because it contributes to overall health and wellness. Discover what external and internal barriers present themselves, and work toward formulating specific goals. This process is ongoing and takes com-mitment and effort. Make an effort to discover activities you and your child prefer, and invest in structuring your time so that effective participation is possible.

Kids and teens now understand:

- The benefits of exercising
- The amount of exercise needed versus the amount of exercise they are currently getting
- The external barriers that may get in the way of participating
- Unhelpful thoughts and rationalizations that may get in the way of participating
- Ways to overcome these thoughts and get motivated to exercise
- How parents can get involved in helping them to participate.

 MINDFULNESS EXERCISE: Getting to the Finish Line

See page 226 for the mindfulness exercise that corresponds to this chapter, and refer to page 217 for instructions on accessing the audio.

10

Getting Others on Board

My parents constantly have candy and snacks all over the house for my younger sister. It makes it impossible for me to try to work on this. It really annoys me, because I tell them how hard it is for me, I get tempted and eat it, and then they get mad at me. —ELLA, AGE 13

I always try to ask for the things I need and teach my kids to be assertive in asking for what they want and need, too. I try to teach my daughter to ask waiters and waitresses in restaurants to make changes to the food they are offering, but she gets too embarrassed and refuses. —EVE, PARENT

EVEN WHEN KIDS AND TEENS have chosen to implement their health goals, they must still be able to communicate these goals to friends, family, and others, such as cafeteria and restaurant staff. In this chapter, kids and teens will learn skills to help effectively express their needs (for example, asking a server for food to be baked instead of fried or for dressing and sauces on the side rather than directly on foods).

Learning these integral life skills increases the chances that your child's needs will be met. Studies have shown that individuals who receive support throughout their health- and weight-management journeys are more likely to succeed and maintain successful behavioral changes for the long term.[154]

I encourage you and your child to seek support from the people your child interacts with to stay accountable and boost motivation throughout the process. In this chapter, you will learn how to seek support. In most cases, you and your child can find healthy alternatives to old habits so that there are fewer barriers leading to self-sabotaging behaviors. Role-playing exercises also teach your child methods of engaging in positive, effective, and empowering interactions.

Going out to eat is an essential time when the 4Ps come in handy (see Chapter 5 for a review of the 4Ps). Teach your child to *predict, plan, put into action, and practice* when challenging situations arise. Last, this chapter provides a general overview of school policies when it comes to food and eating and encourages you and your child to advocate for standards that directly and positively have an impact on your child's health.

TELL IT LIKE IT IS

Review Health Assertiveness

Your child has the right to assert himself and be heard, but there may be thoughts, feelings, or personal characteristics that get in the way of his initiating conversations in order to get his needs met. Your child may be shy by nature or have difficulty with expressive language. He also may be flooded with self-defeating thoughts, such as, "No one will listen to me," "I'm shy so I can't," "I don't know how to express myself," or "_____ will be angry with me if I assert myself." Whatever the case, having a template for effective, assertive communication is essential to guide your child's ability to express his health needs.

Make it a rule of thumb that he make efforts to express himself firmly and respectfully. He should be very clear about what he's asking for, explaining why it would be beneficial to him, and asking directly for support from others.

Note that asking for what he needs comes with the risk that the other person may not react in the way that he wanted or expected them to. That may naturally provoke feelings of sadness, disappointment, frustration, anger, etc., within him. That's okay. Convey to him that he still has the right to live healthfully and not dismiss his own needs. Your child will be more open to taking these risks if he has your support and encouragement.

ASSERTIVENESS

Inform your child of the difference between being passive, aggressive, and assertive, as the goal is for him to be assertive about his health needs.

PASSIVE: Not taking direct action and letting things go; trying to avoid confrontation.

AGGRESSIVE: Using force (verbal or physical), reacting and interacting negatively, causing confrontation. This takes away from self-confidence, self-love, and integrity.

ASSERTIVE: Being proactive and direct, speaking honestly and respectfully, expressing yourself appropriately for the situation, and taking yourself and others into consideration during the interaction. This contributes to self-confidence, self-love, and integrity.

Convey to your child these tips on how to be assertive[155]:

- Remind yourself that your ideas, opinions, and needs are as important as everyone else's.
- Pay attention to what you think, feel, want, and prefer before communicating that to others.
- Make and keep direct eye contact.
- Face the person directly.
- Be aware of your body language and whether it conveys uneasiness (fidgeting, shifting, etc.).
- Use clear "I" statements, starting with "I feel," "I think," "I would like," and "I prefer" ("you" statements sound blaming).
- Use a firm, confident, and calm voice.
- Pace the rate at which you're speaking so it's not too fast or too slow.
- Discuss your needs and feelings clearly, openly, and honestly.
- Avoid tentative responses ("I wonder whether you could . . ." as opposed to "Could you please . . . ?").
- Don't threaten, blame, ridicule, or put down the other person.
- Speak but also listen to the other person.
- Be mindful of choosing an appropriate time and place for your requests.
- Be open to new ways of thinking about yourself, others, and the situation.
- Be open to problem solving and collaborating with others (see Chapter 5 on the 4Ps and problem solving).
- When you are problem solving, use this formula: "I feel . . . when you . . . because. . . . I would like. . . . How do you see it? How can we resolve this?"

For example, let's say your friend is pressuring you to go to your favorite donut shop because she wants to share a donut with you. You decide not to go because you fear this will trigger overeating and that you'll likely share a donut and get another to follow. You can say to your friend, "*I feel uncomfortable when you ask me over and over again to go to the donut shop after I said I'd rather not go, because I made the decision that I don't want a donut right now. I would appreciate and like it if you could hear me the first time I say it. How do you see it? How can we resolve this* so you get what you want, too?"

OBSTACLES TO ASSERTING HEALTH NEEDS[156]

Express to your child that as much as he may prefer it, it is actually virtually impossible to meet all of his health needs alone. There are times that he'll need to assert himself and reach out for support and help. It is important to be selective of whom he asks. He can choose to avoid people who historically judge, criticize, and/or blame him and reach out to those who care and will most likely listen and take action to help him.

Here are common obstacles to assertiveness, and how to overcome them.

1. *Believing that to need and get help is a sign of weakness.* As humans, we are all imperfect, face challenges, and need help. Being able to reach out and ask for what you need is a sign of strength rather than weakness.

2. *Thinking that you don't deserve support and help.* Everyone is deserving of and needs help now and then. We sometimes attach a stigma to asking for support around our health needs. If you needed help reaching something on a high shelf, you may think, *I can't help that I'm short, so it is okay that I need help getting the cereal that's out of my reach.* But with your health needs, you may mistakenly think, *I am to blame for the position I'm in, so why should I ask for help? I'm not deserving of the support and should be able to handle it on my own.*

3. *Not speaking up to ask for help.* As much as you would sometimes appreciate it, no one can read your mind. It's likely that others do not know that you need help and support unless you inform them that you do. You may be masking your emotions or giving off the

impression through body language or your demeanor that you're coping okay or that you don't want support. It is best to be direct and clear.

4. *Giving up too easily.* If support does not come quickly, you may be tempted to give up. Getting help can sometimes take a while, especially if you need to make multiple attempts and requests. Sometimes that has nothing to do with you but rather the other person. They may be busy, preoccupied, or don't know how important it is to you or that you need help immediately.

Ask your child, "What obstacles can you relate to? What may present itself and get in the way of you asserting yourself? How will you handle the challenge?" Role-play the problem-solving formula with a challenging situation he may encounter.

STRATEGY 47

OUT AND ABOUT

Know the Nuances of Eating Out

The US Department of Agriculture estimates that we eat 29 percent of our meals away from home.[157] Going out to eat most likely will be a challenge for your child. It can be a challenge for most of us, because we have less control over the ingredients that go into our meals. If you're looking for healthy food options at a restaurant, it's often necessary to assert yourself and ask for alternatives. At the same time, we often get caught up in rationalizing that we are eating out and are deserving of special treats (see Chapters 4 and 9 on power cards to work through these rationalizations). Also, there's the added pressure of natural temptations—for example, the bread and olive oil in front of us on the table—and the people who share our company may not be mindful of what they're eating.

Eating out is a prime example of when the 4Ps come in handy. Convey to your child that she needs to *predict, plan ahead, put into action, and practice* when she's eating out. Review these tips with her.

PREDICT

- Consider what ordinarily presents as a challenge when you eat out. For example, if you tend to take home leftovers and have a midnight snack of the leftovers, avoid taking leftover food home. Reflect on your history and gauge your level of vulnerability (this can be based on your mood, your self-confidence, etc.) and level of hunger and cravings prior to eating out. Accept that history will probably repeat itself and what might have not worked for you in the past is likely to not work for you now. After identifying potential challenges, plan ahead by using the suggestions below, and make concerted efforts to follow through.

PLAN AHEAD

- Look at an online menu to ensure that you'll have healthy food choices.
- Narrow down healthy options from the online menu to avoid having to make on-the-spot decisions.
- Call ahead and ask about the restaurant's flexibility regarding altering their menu choices to meet your dietary needs (substituting vegetables for french fries, baking or grilling foods instead of frying them, etc.).
- Be aware of foods that can be prepared alternatively or choose to leave out ingredients to suit your needs and taste.
- Avoid going out to eat when you're famished.
- If the restaurant has a buffet option, and that has been an overeating trigger for you in the past, order an item from the menu instead of opting for the all-you-can-eat buffet.

PUT THE PLAN INTO ACTION

- Don't be afraid to ask for healthier choices and/or food alternatives when you are eating out. Restaurants and servers are used to accommodating patrons based on their dietary needs.

193

- It's easy to get tempted by chips, peanuts, Chinese noodles, or a basket of bread. These foods are usually eaten mindlessly, so if you choose to have them, be sure to eat them mindfully.
- Think about where to sit at a table, as appetizers and bread baskets are usually placed in the center of the table.
- Pay attention to portion sizes (see the serving size chart on page 72) and, if needed, plan to take home leftovers.
- Don't feel forced to order from the kids' menu. These typically have less healthful options.
- Consider ordering dishes that are grilled, steamed, boiled, poached, roasted, stir-fried, blackened, or baked, as opposed to buttered, breaded, creamed, scalloped, au gratin, sautéed, pan-fried, or fried.
- Whenever possible, choose red sauce over cream sauce or gravies.
- Try ketchup, mustard, soy sauce, barbecue sauce, salsa, or taco sauce instead of mayonnaise, tartar sauce, or creamy sauces or dips.
- Skip sugary drinks.
- Drink water throughout the meal.
- Ask for salad dressing on the side, use a modest amount on your salad, or ask for a lighter option.
- Be mindful when using dressings and condiments.
- Ask if foods contain butter or margarine—especially vegetables. If they do, suggest cooking them with a little oil or steaming them.
- Ask to go light on the oil, especially for foods that are sautéed.
- Ask if whole-grain bread is available if you choose to have a piece.
- Pace yourself to eat more slowly.
- Refrain from automatically "cleaning your plate." Be mindful of your hunger and fullness cues (see Chapter 1 on mindfulness).
- Ask if dessert alternatives such as berries or assorted fruits are available.
- Opt to share dishes and desserts if the portions are large.
- Throughout the meal, eat slowly and mindfully.

Go online and check out the menu of your child's favorite restaurant. Have your child evaluate the food choices and see if there are lighter options that she can eat or others she would want to alter. Role-play with your child about how you would assert yourself with the server if you were asking for an alternative to an entrée that you wanted to order.

Going out to eat can be a challenge because of all the factors mentioned. If you and your child have an awareness of how to strategize and work through those challenges, you can build up your child's confidence. You'll strengthen her belief that she can persevere through any challenge that comes up and meet her healthful goals. Having an ongoing dialogue about potential challenges that may come up leads to greater awareness, a stronger knowledge base, and a deeper connection with you.

STRATEGY 48

SHOW THE LOVE

Express Your Need for Support

Asking for the support of family, friends, and others your child interacts with can influence the success of long-term healthful changes. It's an effective way of helping your child stay accountable to his goals and can help boost his motivation through the process. But how do you communicate when people may not always understand your challenges? Review these tips and examples with your child to help him express his need for support.

- Have an open dialogue with family members and ask them for support to make the changes that are necessary to help you reach your goals. Let them know what you may need and that you are open to exploring solutions for your health and well-being.
- Let other people know your challenges and ask for assistance in the moment. For example, if you're at a restaurant and you typically overdo it on the bread, feel free to ask that the bread be moved to the opposite side of the table, or ask if it's okay with whomever you are with that the bread be left off the table altogether.

- Sometimes when you reach out for support, you may get more than you bargained for. You may find individuals frequently commenting on the foods you're eating and continually inquiring how your journey is going. That may be okay for some, but if it is overwhelming and unwelcome for you, you can set parameters and indicate specific ways that your friends can be most helpful. They won't know unless you tell them.

- We don't have control over how people react to the choices we make. They may have judgments about these choices, and some may feel free to share their opinions even if their feedback isn't asked for. You can set boundaries and thoughtfully let others know that you have your own opinions you're electing to stick to.

- It can be helpful to anticipate how people's own feelings may influence their reaction to you. For some, your new health regimen may reflect something they would like to be doing but aren't. Or they may have their own ideas about food and health and approach it in an entirely different way. You can respectfully acknowledge where they are coming from while being clear about your own needs.

EXAMPLES OF RESPONSES TO A FAMILY MEMBER

Imagine that even after you've expressed your desire to eat more health-fully, your aunt offers you a brownie she just baked. In the past, you never refused because of wanting her to know how appreciative you are of her kindness and fine baking skills. How might you respond to her?

Some positive responses include:

- "Thanks, I know you made the brownies especially for me, but I'm not really hungry right now."
- "If I ate the brownie now, it would go to waste because I'm too full to enjoy it."
- "Please don't think my refusal means I don't value all the hard work you put into making those brownies."
- "Thank you for understanding, but I can't eat the brownie right now."
- "I appreciate you baking this for me, and it is so hard for me to say no, but I need to at this time."

- Purchasing snack packs as opposed to full bags of snacks, or portioning snacks into snack-size ziplock bags.
- Generally not allowing candy or less-healthy snacks inside the house unless it's portioned out and reserved for certain occasions such as Halloween or birthday parties. Even on these occasions, kids can be mindful about consumption. For example, during Halloween, you can ration out a few candies that can be eaten over the week and donate or give away leftover candy.
- Keeping only small-portion sizes of ice cream, as opposed to a quart or half gallon, on hand at any given time.
- Keeping only low-calorie beverages in the house.
- Always having fresh fruits and vegetables available at home.

EXERCISE: Asking for Support

Have your child role-play a scenario where he needs to ask a family member for support.

- Practice asserting your needs to a family member. You could choose to express a challenge you're having or ask for a specific way your family member can be supportive of your healthful needs.
- Now pretend to be your family member receiving the information.
- Identify how you feel doing the role play from the different points of view (yourself/your family member) and how it feels asserting your need for support.

It helps to get other people on board—with time, they typically accommodate changes and try to be helpful. I fully remember when I transitioned to a healthier lifestyle that it took others time to adjust. Some people were more open to it than others. Over time, most people were thoughtful, helpful, and supportive.

CAFÉ USDA

Advocate for School Food Policies

Is your school a partner in your child's nutrition? Or is it promoting unhealthy choices? Commercials, vending machines, contracts with snack and soft-drink companies, and à la carte foods in schools, as well as the ubiquitous treats at classroom parties, fund-raisers, and other school events, all add up to a major problem in the fight against childhood obesity. Having less-healthful foods readily accessible prompts kids and teens to indulge in them. Who wouldn't, when faced with the choice between french fries and carrot sticks? Let's take a look at the nutritional health standards for schools so you can assess whether your child's school is making the grade.

FEDERAL PROGRAMS

At the federal level, the Healthy, Hunger-Free Kids Act of 2010 required the United States Department of Agriculture (USDA) to establish nutrition standards for all foods sold in schools. The legislation sets policy for the USDA's core child-nutrition programs and establishes standards for federally reimbursable school meals, which include the National School Lunch Program (NSLP) and School Breakfast Program (SBP). Notably, each local school that participates in the NSLP or other federal child nutrition programs is required by law to establish a wellness policy.

The USDA defines foods that are not served as part of the NSLP as "competitive foods" because students might use them to replace healthier foods served as part of the core lunch program.[158] The current regulations for competitive foods, such as those sold à la carte or in vending machines, stipulate that schools prohibit the sale of items of minimal nutritional value during meal periods in the food service area where NSLP meals are sold or eaten.[159]

The USDA "Smart Snacks in School" standards were enacted in the 2014–2015 school year. These are national health guidelines for all school foods, including à la carte options and snacks and beverages in vending machines.[160] For example, snack items should not exceed 200 calories each or contain more than 230 mg of sodium per item. These standards draw on recommendations from the Institute of Medicine, existing voluntary standards already implemented by thousands of schools around the country, and healthy food and beverage offerings already available in the marketplace.[161]

Every five years, the US departments of Health and Human Services (HHS) and Agriculture (USDA) update their dietary guidelines.[162] They recommend water as the beverage of choice: "Strategies are needed to encourage the US population, especially children and adolescents, to drink water when they are thirsty." And, for the first time, the Dietary Guidelines Advisory Committee is recommending that products containing added sugar comprise no more than 10 percent of someone's daily caloric intake. These recommendations are in line with those of the World Health Organization, which actually go a step further by encouraging people to eat no more than 5 percent of daily calories from added sugar.

The committee's sugar recommendations were specifically geared toward kids and teens. They say that there should be more efforts to reduce added sugars in foods and beverages in school meals.

Additionally, the committee says policies are needed that limit exposure to and marketing of foods and beverages high in added sugars to kids, as dietary preferences are established early in life. The average young person views more than three thousand ads per day through television, the Internet, billboards, and magazines.[163] Increasingly, advertisers are targeting younger and younger children in an effort to establish "brand-name preference" at as early an age as possible.[164]

Finally, public education campaigns are needed to increase awareness of the health effects of added sugars and sugar-sweetened beverages and to help consumers reduce their intake. Collectively, all these policies will help improve the health and nutrition of the nation's children, a top priority for the Obama administration.

Future policies should increase subsidies to broaden accessibility of healthy foods in schools and in poor communities. This should be at the forefront for policymakers working to eradicate obesity. Improvements nationwide are unevenly spread, with most happening among more-educated Americans in a higher socioeconomic bracket.

Although American diets improved from 1999 to 2012, with a reduction in trans fats, small increases in fiber, and less soda consumption, most of the advances are not happening among lower-income, less-educated Americans.[165] Poverty and obesity are known to be strongly correlated. When conducting my focus groups for this book, a teen reported walking almost a mile to find a salad to eat for lunch and finally giving up and settling for a hamburger and fries because they were more readily available to him.

WHAT'S GOING ON AT YOUR CHILD'S SCHOOL?

When I interviewed school food services personnel, they reported to me that individual school districts are responsible for enforcing mandated policies, and some are not doing so effectively, especially when it comes to school vending machines. They simply rely on the vendors that are supplying the snacks. In addition, when food is being distributed during school events such as sports, fund-raisers, etc., there is minimal enforcement, and less-healthful snacks are often offered.

Even when relatively healthier snacks are available in school vending machines, some kids are making multiple trips to the vending machines, thereby doubling or tripling their portion sizes. Lastly, the USDA food regulations are not imposed on public schools that opt out of the NSLP or on private schools that are for-profit and are not part of the NSLP; therefore, general food offerings are up to the discretion of these individual schools.

Although the nutritional health of kids and teens at school is now being prioritized more widely, it is important to recognize that when less-healthful foods are available at school, kids will eat them. They will consume foods with more fat and sugar and fewer of the healthier foods such as fruits, vegetables, and milk.[166] The availability of healthful foods in schools is one priority; another should be requiring nutrition education throughout the middle school and high school years. Kids have a greater chance of making more healthful, mindful choices if they are effectively taught about nutrition, how food affects the body, and how their thoughts and impulses influence their actions.

EXERCISE: Review School Policies

If your child's school is part of the NSLP, depending on her age, your child may be aware that school policies have recently changed to include more healthful foods and snacks. Review the policies with her (the websites are available in Resources, page 248), and ask her to observe and respond to:

- Whether your school is abiding by the policies set by the USDA
- Any reactions to these policy changes

- If having restrictions over food at school is helpful in meeting your healthful goals and behaviors
- If you and others are eating more healthfully and mindfully outside of school.

If your child's school opted out of the NSLP or she attends a private school, ask her to observe:

- Whether any nutritional changes were made over the last several years and what they were
- What other changes you think would be helpful in helping to eat more healthfully at school
- Whether during your school day you're offered more healthful food or snack options.

Ask your child what nutritional education she has received at school. Discuss what changes she would like to see made at her school. Getting kids actively interested in their health not only promotes personal responsibility but also boosts their motivation to make positive changes to their eating behaviors.

CHECK YOUR BAGGAGE

What if you have personal challenges with asserting yourself and setting appropriate boundaries? Be aware of how you approach your child. Encouraging your child is an important part of this process. You can effectively help your child even if you yourself experience negative, self-defeating thoughts or need to improve your ability to effectively assert yourself. By modeling effective behaviors for your child, you can simultaneously experience personal growth through the process.

When you go through the techniques, apply them to yourself, too. You can reassure your child about obstacles that may come up and share your own challenges, as well. These discussions can help you learn about facets of your child that you may not have known previously.

Going out to eat may be an ideal time to discuss and practice new skills together. Of course, helping your child express the need for support may also evoke uncomfortable thoughts or feelings for you. So be open to challenging yourself and looking at things more expansively. Try considering all options or doing things differently than you may have in the past.

You may or may not be aware of how certain policies or regulations affect your child's access to certain foods at school. Exploring this with your child is helpful because your child needs to take personal responsibility for healthful behavior. Asserting those needs and possibly advocating for changes is a direct action that your child can take.

 REVIEW

Teaching kids and teens to identify and assert their needs and set their own boundaries is essential as they become aware that no one can read their minds. Even if parents help guide behavior, there is still a need for kids and teens to independently practice communication, assertiveness, and problem-solving skills. These are crucial skills for independent living. It's also important to gain awareness of potential barriers that may get in the way.

Kids and teens should know:

- Why being assertive is so critical
- The difference between passive, aggressive, and assertive communication
- Specific assertiveness techniques
- Obstacles to asserting healthful needs
- The challenges that may come up when going out to eat
- How to apply the 4Ps when going out to eat
- Tips for eating healthily while eating out
- Ways to express the need for support
- How to respond to a family member with positive communication
- How to get support at home
- Policies and standards that may impact access to healthy food at school.

 MINDFULNESS EXERCISE: The Sunset from the Mountaintop

See page 227 for the mindfulness exercise that corresponds to this chapter, and refer to page 217 for instructions on accessing the audio.

Guiding Kids and Teens to Get Back on Track

I still have those moments when I overeat or go a few days when I don't exercise. It doesn't happen all that often, but it still makes me feel disappointed in myself. Will I ever get this right?

—SILVIE, AGE 18

My son has really made a change, and I'm so proud of him. He has lost 15 pounds, but I'm fearful he'll gain it back, because I still see him overeating at times. I feel the urge to jump in and say something, but I hold back. It's not easy.

—ROBIN, PARENT

DETOURS ON THE ROAD to better health are normal—they happen to everyone. Slipping up is being human and does not have to lead to giving up on a healthy practice. By being able to continue to take action steps even if kids have had a tough day or week, they can still gain mastery over their eating and exercise goals.

As kids and teens evolve, they will learn to "get back on the horse" when the inevitable slips occur. They'll identify strategies for slips that focus on their attitude, thoughts, and actions. This chapter teaches them to internalize their beliefs so that they can be successful at their healthful goals and that they have the power to make choices.

First, kids and teens must be able to differentiate between "slipping" and "falling." It's important for them to know that they can control whether an event is a *slip*, which is temporary, or a *fall*, which is a prolonged return to old behavior patterns that negatively impact their health.

This chapter includes tips for having a more positive attitude and the steps to take after a slipup. In the process, your child will learn to expect challenges, focus on how your child went down a certain path, and understand what triggers and "stinking thinking" were operating. By learning problem-solving skills, your child will build confidence and be more inspired to return to working on values and goals.

"I'VE SLIPPED AND I CAN'T GET UP"

Gain Perspective on Setbacks

Your child's mind will easily go to the place of evaluating whether he's doing his healthy practice "right" or "wrong." His mind will further loop to suggest that when he's doing it "wrong," then he's doing poorly, is therefore ineffective, and will probably never get it right. He may be convinced that he needs to get the behavior right all the time. This is reflective of all-or-nothing, black-and-white thinking (see Chapter 4 on stinking thinking). He may fear that he'll forget the skills, be frustrated that he can't follow them all the time, or be concerned that he'll return to unhealthy past eating and exercise behaviors and feel like a failure.

It's important to stress that no one is perfect. There is always room for slips, refocusing, and recalibrating. Your child will inevitably have days when eating right is effortless and days when it's more difficult for him. *It's the overall picture that matters most.* Over time, is he able to be generally consistent and committed? Inevitably, it is he who gets to focus on when he's hungry and thirsty and decide what he wants to eat and drink and how much. He can mindfully choose to have a piece of cake instead of impulsively and mindlessly eating it. If he eats it mindfully, he'll be left feeling proud that he stuck to his plan and chose to have one piece rather than two pieces of cake, or changed his plan to eat sorbet and fruit salad instead of cake. If he eats the cake impulsively, he may experience shame and disappointment because his behavior was led purely by his self-sabotaging thoughts rather than by his values.

Consider the adversity your child faces on a daily basis. For one, he needs to eat (he cannot practice abstinence) and will always be exposed to triggers and situations that can potentially be challenging for him. His brain's reward center still wants the dopamine release that some foods trigger; it won't stop "wanting" even if he makes a philosophical change to how he approaches eating and exercise behaviors. He will still have ongoing responses to food, eating, and exercise, as well as self-defeating

204

thoughts and feelings, which he will continually need to work through. Maintaining a healthy practice requires acceptance of all of this and an understanding that at times these vulnerabilities will make it harder to stick to the plan.

The practice of living a healthy life always has what may feel like setbacks. Slips are expected and inevitable. They need to be put into perspective and worked through so that a challenging day or week does not become challenging weeks and months. Typically, the longer that the slip lasts, the greater the chance that kids and teens will feel hopeless and decide to give up healthy practices.

To illustrate the need to persist through adversity, use the example of climbing a mountain with your child. While climbing a steep mountain, your child becomes tired and discouraged (a perceived setback), and, rather than climbing all the way down, he takes a rest, hydrates, reminds himself why the climb is meaningful for him, and recalibrates. He continues to climb the mountain and accomplishes what he set out to do with the understanding that more challenges may come up along the way.

Like any good practice, skills and habits are built one day at a time. With commitment and effort, even if your child had a particularly challenging day, he can rebound and focus on getting back on track. Review with your child these tips about slips.

Gaining Perspective on Slipups

- Slips are inevitable. Expect them to happen.
- To diminish the potential for avoidance, procrastination, and self-defeating thoughts, it is best to try to get back on track as soon as you possibly can after a slip.
- A slip is not a sign of failure. We all slip, which is a characteristic of our being human. Instead, it is a temporary setback amidst a difficult challenge.
- No slip can erase all your healthful progress.
- You can always rebound from a slip.
- You can always learn something valuable about yourself from a slip. Think about it as an opportunity to do so.
- Use a slip as a signal that you are in need of additional support—seek and be accepting of it.
- You may get discouraged and frustrated at times, especially during a slip. These are typical feelings. In any given moment,

try to accept whatever comes up. They are only thoughts and feelings. They do not dictate what you *do* with the thoughts and feelings. You can feel discouraged *and* still get back on track.

* The best thing you can do is to understand the slips so they can be avoided or worked through effectively in the future.

STRATEGY 51

SLIPPERY SITUATIONS

What to Do During and After Slips

The goal is for kids and teens to develop the necessary skills to face daily eating and exercise challenges. Then they will be able to predict situations that may arise and be ready for any circumstance. With this mental shift comes self-assurance and a more positive attitude, and kids will be able to take action from a place of openness, self-acceptance, and self-compassion. These skills can be applied not only to health goals but also to other life challenges that surface.

Kids and teens often feel like throwing in the towel after a slipup because of the mistaken perception that they will never succeed. But if it's thought of rationally, will progress be greatly affected by one or two meals where a kid slips into old behavior habits? No. When kids decide to stick to their health goals despite a setback, they give themselves the opportunity to repair the notion that "they are not good at it, so why bother trying?" All is not lost, and there is always a choice to get back on track quickly.

If and when your child slips, self-criticism is likely to surface, and those feelings will not help her regain the control she feels she lost. They can erode her self-confidence when she needs it most. These thoughts can be reframed as, "I'm having the thought that I'm not good at it," as opposed to "I'm buying into the belief that I'm not good at it," or "I have the thought that I'm not good at it, but I'm choosing to still try my best and accept that I won't be perfect. When I'm not, all is not lost, and I can be proud of my accomplishments."

When she has particularly negative thoughts regarding herself, challenge her by asking these two questions:

1. What is a more useful or helpful way of looking at this?

2. If a friend described the same situation and reaction, what advice would you give to him? How would you treat him? You would probably be calm, supportive, and kind. Apply those loving-kindness sentiments to yourself.

Then, have your child assess the situation. Was the overeating due to any of the challenges below? Or some others?

1. **AN EMOTIONAL RESPONSE, WHETHER POSITIVE OR NEGATIVE, TO A SITUATION:** For example, you're feeling disappointed because you "messed up" the presentation you made in front of the class at school.

2. **A BREAK IN DAILY ROUTINE:** For example, you went on vacation, you're eating out practically every meal, and it's hard to fit in exercising.

3. **A HEIGHTENED PHYSIOLOGICAL STATE:** For example, you feel elated, your heart is racing in excitement, and you want to "fully" celebrate your team's victory.

4. **CONFRONTING AN INTENSE CRAVING OR URGE:** For example, you go to a friend's house, and he unexpectedly serves your favorite ice cream.

Taking an inventory of both the negative thinking and what was challenging about a given situation can help your child gain awareness about what causes her slips. This in turn will enable her to continue to make progress so that the slips are less frequent and so that she is less inclined to feel discouraged, ashamed, and hopeless. She will have a better sense of how to handle slips more effectively.

EXERCISE: Identify the Triggers

Here's a step-by-step way for your child to more clearly identify what caused a slipup. Ask her to analyze a recent slipup by asking the following questions:

1. What circumstance led to the slip? (e.g., I went to the movies and then had dinner at a friend's house and ate a lot more chips and popcorn than I wanted to. The following day I continued eating more chips at home when the neighbors came over.)

2. What were you thinking before, during, and after the slip? (e.g., Before: I haven't had these snacks in a long time; I'll stop at a handful. During: This is too hard. After: I'll never be able to do this.)

3. How were you feeling? (e.g., Before: Frustrated and irritated. During: Out of control and frenzied. After: Disappointed in myself and ashamed about the behavior.)

4. How did you react? (e.g., I ate many handfuls of popcorn, pretzels, and corn chips over a two-day period.)

5. What else could you have done in those circumstances? (e.g., I could have problem solved through it [see Chapter 5] and decided not to take any, or I could have mindfully had a certain portion of each snack.)

6. What resources/supports need to be in place in order for you to react differently? (e.g., I could have looked for vegetables, asked if there were any healthier snacks, or even asked my friend to gently remind me if I was eating more than I intended to. I could have recognized that I was triggered and taken notice of it for the next day.)

7. Are you noticing any pattern(s) with your slips? (e.g., They happen during social situations, particularly when I'm feeling worried.)

Every slip is a learning opportunity and enhances your child's self-awareness and ability to problem solve. She is learning to track her patterns of thoughts, feelings, and behaviors before, during, and after a slip. She is practicing working through challenging situations to get back to her values of healthful living.

SPEEDY RECOVERY

Eight Steps to Break the Slip-Fall Cycle

You want your child to recover quickly from a slip so that it doesn't snowball into a full-fledged fall that would be more challenging to rebound from. You could provide him with this example: If you're running and you feel your pain in your heel, it's often better to sit out the race than to struggle and worsen your injury. The initial injury (grade 1) can result in approximately a one-week rest period, whereas a significant injury (grade 3) can result in a month or longer rest period. The longer and more significant the fall, the harder it can be to rebound from it. It's best to try to avoid that pattern and learn to quickly get back on track.

EXERCISE: The Slip-Fall Pattern

Outline the following pattern for your child and then ask him to practice the eight steps that follow to break the slip-fall cycle.

> Challenging Situation ➔ No Plan or Difficulty Accessing Current Plan to Handle It ➔ *Slip* ➔ Negative Thinking and Self-Talk ➔ Discouraging, Shameful, and Hopeless Feelings ➔ *Continue to Slip* ➔ More Intense Negative Thinking and Uncomfortable Feelings ➔ *Fall*

EIGHT STEPS TO BREAK THE SLIP-FALL CYCLE

STEP 1: Recognize that no matter how you may feel after the slip, it's not unusual for this to happen. Be open to seizing the learning opportunity.

STEP 2: Identify the negative thoughts and uncomfortable feelings that may lead you to a fall rather than getting you back on track toward your healthful goals. For example, you are probably engaging in all-or-nothing thinking, such as, "I'm *never* going to be able to do this" or, "What's the point? This will *always* be a problem." You may think, "I might as well give up," and end up intensely discouraged.

These are self-sabotaging, exaggerated thoughts that can lead you to spiral, prolong the slip, or prompt you toward a fall. Put these thoughts into perspective. Realize that you are generally successful at this. Slipping is *sometimes* a problem but is not a problem *all* the time. Actually, over time, behavior changes become less strenuous and more habitual and manageable.

STEP 3: Even if you're tempted to give up, allow room for having those thoughts and feelings. Keep moving toward your values and goals while avoiding putting yourself down, even if you aren't feeling successful at the moment. Encourage yourself by pointing out moments of success and notable progress and by proactively doing something toward healthful eating and exercise behaviors.

STEP 4: Evaluate the situation. Reconsider the plan you had in place and whether you need to make adjustments. For example, was the overeating trigger a cluster of issues that came up all at once, such as a misunderstanding with a friend, academic stress, and an argument with your parent? Consider: What was challenging about the situation? Is it likely to happen again? What would you consider doing differently the next time?

STEP 5: Reconnect with your values and goals (review Chapter 2). Remind yourself what your specific values are, why connecting to them is so important to you, the effects that unhealthful behaviors had on you, and how you're going to recommit to your goals.

STEP 6: Problem solve through the challenge (review Chapter 5). Commit to making at least two small changes in the moment. Do something proactive right away to build confidence and show that you can and will do something for your health.

STEP 7: Develop a concrete plan for handling "slippery" situations. For example, have him write down:

I find myself in slippery situations when _____
_____. The plan I will put into place includes:
_____.

STEP 8: Seek support and check in with yourself on a daily and weekly basis to acknowledge your accomplishments and assess your progress.

Long-term weight and health management is significantly more effective when problem-solving mechanisms are in place.[167]

STRATEGY 53

RECONNECT WITH YOUR BEST SELF

Empower Kids and Teens to Forge Ahead

The coping strategy your child is using to work through food issues such as cravings, emotional eating, etc., affects her long-term weight maintenance. It's not enough to learn new behaviors and reinforce "good" behaviors by imposing consequences on negative ones. Kids also need to overcome the psychological barriers that have an impact on behaviors. There are many studies that show that a combination of cognitive and mindfulness approaches help long-term effectiveness.[168] Now, we will integrate a mind-body approach.[169] This way, your child will best be able to accept challenging situations as they arise and have the flexibility to work through them.[170]

EXERCISE: Reconnecting with Your Best You Following a Slip

Encouraging your child to write a guided journal entry, as follows, after a slip integrates new perspectives, which will help her adopt healthier behaviors. She has the opportunity to look at what triggered the behavior, assess and accept what happened, including negative and uncomfortable thoughts and feelings, identify what she could learn for future circumstances, and encourage herself to do it differently next time—so that she can be her "best me."

The challenging situation was _____

_____

I am vulnerable to slips in my eating when _____

_____

I am vulnerable to slips in my exercising when _____

_____

Yes, I slipped and feel _____ at the moment; however, I also want to remember my past successes, which include

_____

I'm going to notice my negative thoughts and feelings about myself and about the situation. Instead of giving up and letting it affect me even more, I choose to take control and get back on track. I'm going to do that now by doing the following things: _____

_____

I'm going to do these things even though I'm thinking and feeling
_____. I
know that this is a typical part of the process. I'm going to take the moment to learn about my behaviors. What I learned from this experience about my eating and exercising includes:

_____

These points are going to help me so that I slip less often. I care about being my best me, and I am committed to continue working on my health goals. *Anything I want to be successful at, I need to commit to working at.* I will embrace and be mindful of this mantra.

Much of what will help kids and teens work through daily weight-management challenges is their ability to effectively problem solve. Problem-solving methods will help them effectively predict, prepare, and plan for challenges that are both health related and beyond.

Sticking with healthy goals definitely takes effort; however, the rewards of reaching a level of accomplishment are boundless. And all is not lost because of a setback. Just as if your child did poorly on an individual math test, the course grade for the quarter is not necessarily dictated by that one particular grade. She could put concerted effort in, work hard to excel for the next exam and beyond, and overall do well in the course.

As kids and teens continue to put effort into their health, healthful habits become a natural part of their lifestyle. They end up with the added benefits of thinking more positively, feeling better, and becoming substantially more confident in themselves. It is important that they realize that if they slip or fall, they can't change the past, but there's always an opportunity to get back on track and create their own present and future. It is never too late to improve. There is always room for growth at any age and at any time, now and throughout their lives.

▮▮▮ CHECK YOUR BAGGAGE

You may be able to relate to the slip-and-fall cycle of getting off track, as most of us do. It is what keeps most people from maintaining a healthful practice for the long term. Some parents assume that they can't teach their children if they don't have it down pat themselves. The fact is that everyone has slips, and no one is perfect at any behavior. Nonetheless, we can still function well, maintain our values, and work toward our goals. You can be effective at guiding your child simply because already know this, because you care, and because you will make the effort to do so.

Convey to your child that it is the big picture that matters most. There's an 80/20 rule to healthy eating: If you're practicing 80 percent of the time in a given week, you'll be able to maintain the benefits of healthy eating you've already achieved. There's no expectation of perfection; it's just not realistic. You can work with your child to practice their new skills and comment on the frustration you sometimes feel, as well. This normalizes your child's thoughts and feelings, and your child will feel supported.

You may also be fearful of your child's slips. You may think to yourself, "Here we go again," "Can't he get this right?" or, "She'll never be able to get this; she's too lazy." Although you may feel guilty for judging your child, it's important to gain self-awareness and inwardly own up to those thoughts and feelings and acknowledge that they may exist for you. With self-awareness and acknowledgment, there's less of a chance that your negativity will trickle into your reactions to and interactions with your child.

You may sometimes struggle with your child's challenges, as many parents do, because you experience them as reflecting on you. You may perceive this struggle as a result of your good or bad teaching or as a representation of you and your family, or it may painfully remind you of attributes you dislike in either another person or yourself. All these reactions are typical for a parent. Just because you are having that perception and reaction does not mean that you will choose to act on it. You get to make that choice.

Another challenge that may come up is the realization of the level of effort and commitment this healthy new practice takes. What's helpful about ongoing practice is that over time the behaviors become habitual and part of your routine like everything else—washing up before bed, showering, or anything else that is an ongoing practice.

Your child will learn to break down a situation and effectively evaluate a slip. You may find yourself thinking, "Why do we need to analyze everything?" To make long-standing changes that stick, your child needs to learn to effectively and independently problem solve. You are guiding your child through this process, and because it takes time to learn and integrate a healthy new practice, initially it is appropriate and helpful to analyze things in such a detailed and thorough way. You now have a step-by-step process that you can walk your child through.

 REVIEW

We discussed the difference between slipping and falling. Parents should help kids and teens work through a slip that can prevent them from following through on their healthful goals. Parents can help guide kids and teens if and when a slip occurs to avoid falling. If the slip-and-fall cycle occurs and old behavior patterns return, parents can help them get back on track no matter how long it's been. This chapter provided specific steps to break the cycle. Kids and teens should reconnect with being the best they can possibly be.

Kids and teens should:

- Understand the difference between a slip and a fall.
- Identify that the overall picture matters the most.
- Identify when certain thoughts and feelings come up before, during, and after a slip.
- Process a slip so that future behaviors can be thoughtful and mindful.
- Stay positive when they slip.
- Recognize a potential slip-fall pattern.
- Work through the eight steps to break the slip-fall cycle.
- Write a journal entry that will reconnect them to be the best they can possibly be.

 MINDFULNESS EXERCISE: You Hold the Power

See page 228 for the mindfulness exercise that corresponds to this chapter, and refer to page 217 for instructions on accessing the audio.

EPILOGUE

YOU HAVE GREAT REASON to feel accomplished and proud. You've taken the time and effort to help your child work toward achieving healthful behaviors. This determination and care is not something to be taken lightly!

As you've seen, we all get caught up in our thinking, for better or for worse. Thoughts can lead kids and teens to great success in regard to their health but can possibly sabotage them, too. Still, thoughts and feelings are not facts—they are something children have rather than who they are. They get to personally decide how they want to act in regard to their values.

In this process, you and your child committed to being present; connecting to core values; getting to know thoughts, feelings, and behaviors related to eating and exercising; using the 4Ps; and learning assertiveness and problem-solving skills. Sticking with a healthy practice and putting continual effort into it is most definitely work; however, the rewards for your child are boundless. Your child will benefit from healthful eating and exercise behaviors, physically feeling better and having increased confidence in the ability to maintain a healthy practice.

Healthy eating is a continual practice, just like anything else worth doing. For example, if your child were interested in taking up ice hockey or figure skating, initially, your child would lack confidence in their skating abilities. Your child might be so off balance that they would regularly stumble and fall on the ice.

For some kids, that would be the end of the road. One child might quit because of the perception that they failed and draw the conclusion that they were a terrible skater. Another might believe they won't ever improve, so there's no point in continuing to learn. Either way, they might be left feeling defeated and disappointed, deny themselves the opportunity to do something they really desired, and feel frustrated that they cannot participate in a sport many of their friends enjoy.

Other kids will stick with it, despite the frustrations that may come up. As they continue to invest their time and energy, they experience disappointment and frustration much less often. Soon, they have improved so much that they are able to learn specific ice hockey and figure skating skills and techniques. They notice their confidence building. They have something to look forward to. They feel skillful and gratified!

When it comes to healthy eating and exercise, your child has the chance to contemplate and choose which person your child would rather be. The person who sticks it out—who decides to stay with it despite any setbacks, frustrations, and disappointments—is left feeling confident and proud, recognizing that the result is worth all the effort! I encourage you and your child to continue being as wonderful as you are, put meaningful effort into working on the strategies in this book, and always *practice, practice, practice*!

> "The curious paradox is that when I accept myself
> just as I am, then I can change."
> —CARL ROGERS

MINDFULNESS EXERCISES

THESE MINDFULNESS EXERCISES HELP you pay attention *fully* in the moment, without judgment. Mindfulness improves your focus, concentration, and responses so that you become more thoughtful when you make choices regarding your health. It also helps to increase your general self-awareness and self-confidence.

You can complete these guided visualization and imagery exercises with your child, or your child can practice them independently. The exercises help integrate and reinforce the skills presented in each chapter, so you can perform them following the chapter or as you are practicing the strategies throughout the chapter. Mindfulness practice provides the most benefit when done daily and consistently. You and your child can decide what is most feasible and beneficial. The exercises should take an average of five minutes each and are designed to be listened to following each chapter. They can be accessed at **michellemaidenberg.com/freeyourchildfromovereating**. The scripts are provided here for your reference.

Use these guidelines to prepare yourself for each mindfulness exercise.

- Get into a comfortable position in your seat.
- Sit upright with a straight posture, feet flat on the floor.
- Rest your hands gently on your knees with palms up or down.
- Close your eyes. (If closing your eyes is too uncomfortable, you can participate with open eyes).
- Take a minute to let your mind settle before you begin the mindfulness exercise.
- After the exercise, take a minute to just sit in silence before opening your eyes or going about your activities.

Being Open to Mind and Body

Sit comfortably and gently close your eyes.

Become aware of your chest inflating and deflating. Your chest is rising, then coming down. As you try to focus on your breath, you may notice that your mind takes you somewhere else. You may be thinking about the day, things you need to accomplish, or challenges you want to work through. If your mind wanders, gently bring it back to your breath and label it "thinking." Do so in a loving, nonjudgmental way. Everyone has mind clutter, but this is the time to focus on yourself and your body.

When you return to your breath, you may find that your mind keeps bringing you back to other thoughts. Again and again, if your mind clutter comes up, gently, nonjudgmentally, and thoughtfully thank your mind for reminding you that it's there and return to your breath. Bring patience, compassion, and care to your mind for its persistence.

As you sit, become aware of your body, physical sensations, feelings of pleasure, and possibly tension. Acknowledge these sensations. Make room for them in every part of you. Let them be—without judgment, without wanting to rid yourself of them. Let them have space in your overall experience.

Notice any sensation, comfortable or uncomfortable, with curiosity and inquisitiveness. Give it space and allow it to be there. Accept all of you and everything you bring to the experience. Thoughts may keep coming up—general thoughts, thoughts about thoughts, and judgment about your thoughts. Remember: Label it "thinking" and come back to your breath.

If you notice a certain quality about your thoughts, if they are in sync with the way you usually think, label that, as well. If you are worrying, label it "worry." If you are feeling angry, label it "anger." If you are judging, label it "judging." If you are planning, label it "planning." Whatever thought arises, gently label it. Just observe it and find yourself with an open heart for your thoughts and for all that you are. Return to your breath.

Your feelings, sensations, and focus may change from moment to moment. Allow yourself to experience it all with an open heart. Allow yourself to be who you are, thinking as you think and feeling as you feel. All breaths and sensations are thriving, wonderful parts of you. All thoughts and feelings are greeted with loving kindness and gratitude as they ebb and flow. Allow them to be, allow yourself to be, just as you are—wonderful, kind, thoughtful, and loving.

Congratulate yourself for your willingness and openness toward your journey.

CHAPTER 2.

Who You Want to Be

Sit comfortably and gently close your eyes.

Feel the stillness, the quiet, the absence of movement. You are noticing you and all that you are. You are here with your body, your mind, your physical sensations, and all the thoughts that come and go. Pay attention to it all and recognize it for what it is. It is a moment in time. You are creating a meaningful moment when you get to focus on you.

Ponder what is meaningful to you: what drives you, what moves you, what compels you, and what your passions are. Ask yourself, who do I want to be? How do I want to represent myself, and what do I want to be remembered for?

Allow those thoughts to soak in. Feel empowered by them. You have the ability to choose who you want to be. If you put in concerted effort, you can be all that you want to be. No force can stop you. You are capable, you are strong, you are viable, and you are powerful. Your essence is durable, solid, and resilient. You can also choose to be flexible, adjustable, and accommodating. You get to decide. You get to create your present and future.

You are spirited, with so many passions for yourself, others, and the world around you. Think about what you want that may also move others and the world. You have the ability to create change. Make a difference in the way that you choose to live. It is up to you. Follow your passions in a meaningful way. You and only you are in the driver's seat, dictating what journey you take and how you will get there.

It is a moment in time: a meaningful moment when you get to focus on all that you are and all you want to be. You get to be driven by your passions and your love and admiration for yourself, others, and the world around you. Your values define you; your actions lead you. Go toward who you want to be. Take that step and leap into a world that you can call your own.

Congratulate yourself for your willingness and openness toward your journey.

Sit comfortably and gently close your eyes.

Allow your thoughts to flow freely and just observe them as they drift. They may wander, they may be contemplative, and they may be imagining. All the while, notice your breath. Notice the breath going in and out of your lungs and your body being comforted by your breath. Keep going back to your breath even if your mind drifts away. Return to your awareness and consciousness.

Imagine yourself jumping aboard a cloud. You are free to roam around it without the consequences of falling off. You can explore all of it. You notice its shape continually changing and evolving. You are mesmerized by its beauty and intensity. You are fascinated by its components, its swirls, its versatility, and the idea that it builds momentum as it flows through the sky.

You decide to embark on a journey. You want to explore all of the cloud and witness all that it does. You decide to take this journey from two points of view—from the perspective of the cloud and from your own perspective.

As you enter the stratosphere, you pass over the earth and its various geographies, cultures, and conditions. You transmit deep empathy, care, and loving kindness for all creatures, all circumstances, and all conditions.

You acknowledge the cloud and the challenges it has to witness on a daily basis. As you transmit empathy, care, and loving kindness to the cloud, you realize that you, too, are in need of empathy, compassion, and acknowledgment of your bravery and all that you are.

You open yourself up to risk, to challenge, and to discomfort, even though you're compelled to do otherwise. You do it because of your desire to grow and change and live a meaningful life. Your bravery leads you to commit to a valued life with empathy, care, and loving kindness for yourself and others.

You are appreciated for your bravery and for living a valued life. You are embraced for it and are shown love by someone you deeply care about. You feel their support, warmth, and comfort. You cherish the moment by taking in their hug fully and intentionally. You hold on to it until the very last moment that you are able to. It is one you want to commit to memory.

You breathe deeply. You focus on your breath, which is a reminder of the support and warmth you have access to when you experience adversity or exasperation. The support is never far away. You can draw upon it whenever you need it. It's yours forever to rely on. You are and forever will be cherished, cared about, and loved. You will never be alone.

Congratulate yourself for your willingness and openness toward your journey.

CHAPTER 4.

Accepting Yourself

Sit comfortably and gently close your eyes.

Recognize thoughts of self-criticism and negative self-talk. Bring your attention to them, what they are saying, and how it feels to have them. Experience what it feels like in your body. Scan your body for sensations of numbness or tension or tingling. Accept these without judgment or criticism. If it is uncomfortable, label it as "uncomfortable." If it is worry, label it as "just worrying." Accept that the thoughts and feelings are temporary, that they will pass, and that you are, in fact, okay and safe.

Accept that negative thoughts and feelings are just that and hold only the meaning that you attach to them. Recite to yourself, "I am at peace with myself. I appreciate who I am. All people have value, and I am a valuable human being. I accept the person I am.

"I accept my challenges. I accept my strengths. I view my challenges as strengths not yet developed, rather than weaknesses. I do not have to be perfect to be an okay person. I am perfectly all right just the way I am. I recognize that I am different from others, not better or worse, just different. I slip just like everyone because I am human. I accept my humanness. I embrace my humanness. I celebrate my humanness.

"I will continue to be compassionate, kind, thoughtful, attentive, and generous toward myself, as I want people to be toward me and as I want to be toward others."

Say to yourself: "May I be well; may I accept myself; may I be peaceful. May I be patient, may I have courage, and may I have the understanding and determination to work through challenges, because I am capable and worthy."

Allow for positive self-sentiments to envelop you. Recognize that you are unique. You are powerful. You are wonderful. You are you.

Congratulate yourself for your willingness and openness toward your journey.

Striving for What You Want

Sit comfortably and gently close your eyes.

Settle into your posture with your back upright. Allow yourself to be right here in the moment. Be here exactly as you are. Be exactly who you are. Everything about you is kind and loving.

Notice your breath as it enters and exits your lungs—simple and easy breaths, inhaling and exhaling. Peacefully, quietly, and compassionately notice your body and notice your breath. Notice all that's coming up for you. Sit with awareness of your body, all aspects of it. Notice your mood and how you feel, without judgment. Just as it is.

Think about something you want: something you strive for and yearn for. Have something specific in mind: something you think endlessly about because it is meaningful to you. As you think about what you want, without judgment, notice the thoughts and feelings that are coming up, peacefully, quietly, and compassionately. Think about why this is so important to you. Contemplate what drives the desire you have for it. Notice how your body feels when you connect with this strong desire and passion. Notice where you feel it in your body.

Think about what you need to do to get what you want. Trust in yourself and in your abilities. Imagine fully believing in yourself. You are capable, you are powerful, and you can accomplish anything you want to. Imagine yourself feeling strong and empowered, because you strived and worked for what you wanted, and got it.

You feel accomplished, wholly, deeply, and meaningfully. Connect with the feeling as it is happening in the moment. You feel gratitude in your body and mind because your desire has turned into a reality that you can celebrate. Your posture is upright and tall because you feel proud and dignified in your accomplishment.

Savor who you are. You are okay with just being you, because you are wonderful. Everything about you is kind and loving. You feel proud for all that you are, all that you have accomplished, and all that you will accomplish in the present and in the future. Notice your breath as it enters and exits your lungs. They are simple, easy, and relaxed breaths. You are inhaling and exhaling slowly, peacefully, quietly, and compassionately. Notice your body and notice your breath. Be proud of all you are and all you strive for. You are wonderful, you are driven, and you are accomplished.

Congratulate yourself for your willingness and openness toward your journey.

CHAPTER 6.

You Are Who You Are

Sit comfortably and gently close your eyes.

Plant your feet on the floor and notice the ground beneath you. Notice the feeling in your feet and the security of being able to feel the floor. You are here in the present moment. Your body is slowly relaxing in your seat.

Imagine yourself as a leaf slowly flowing down a river, ebbing and flowing with the current below you. Your body moves tenderly in the direction of the current. You feel whisked away and pick up speed as the current grows stronger. It feels so freeing, and you notice the abundance of energy and movement that surrounds and provides you with comfort and momentum.

Notice the different leaves you pass on your journey. Appreciate all the beauty and robust colors—the essence of each, appreciating each for its own uniqueness. Notice the elements you share with them, the oneness, universality, and connection you feel. Sit with all your varying thoughts and feelings as you continue to steadily flow down the river.

Feel the flow and take in the sensations as you embrace nature and all that you have to offer to this world. Take a deep breath. Notice that you are who you are, with all of your beauty and graciousness. Notice the vast world and all that it has to offer you. You can have it all and know how to make that happen for yourself. You take the journey in the direction you choose. You have the power to go where you want to and be all that you choose to be. You and only you hold that power. Go in the direction of your heart and toward being the best you can be.

Congratulate yourself for your willingness and openness toward your journey.

Sit comfortably and gently close your eyes.

Plant your feet on the floor and notice the ground beneath you. Notice the feeling in your feet and the security of being able to feel the floor. Notice your breath and how it moves in your lungs. Notice the inhalation and the exhalation, how the air flows deeply in and out. Notice your thoughts and feelings—just notice it all.

Visualize that you're a vibrant bird. At first, you're having difficulty allowing your wings to flow freely through all the beauty that surrounds you. Your body fails you, and you feel exasperated by the struggle. You yearn to be free and independent, soaring through the air.

Take a moment to be still and relax your body in hopes that you will be able to be with what is, the predicament you find yourself in. Continue to dream of what could be and all that you can be a part of if given the chance.

Finally, your wings open. You suddenly feel a surge of energy, hopefulness, and excitement. The exhilaration of being able to fly and show yourself as you are is more than you could ever imagine. You feel warmth, connection, and serenity with nature. You soar through the air without hesitation. You are at peace.

You can freely explore the boundaries of this earth with all your glory. You feel the wind rippling around your body, awakening your spirit, and reminding you how grateful you are for being able to be.

You are delighted by everything you see; each and every tree, meadow, lake, and mountainside enchants you. You marvel at it all. You thank the world for all that it is and thank yourself for being all that you are. You are whole and free to soar. The world awaits you. Go out there and try your best to achieve all that you want to. Do everything in your power to live a life you enjoy and feel proud of. Each and every step you take is an important one and gets you closer to the life you want. Take that step now. Go soar.

Congratulate yourself for your willingness and openness toward your journey.

Awareness of Your Body

Sit comfortably and gently close your eyes.

Pause and notice your body. Pay attention to all the feelings and sensations. Notice the comfortable sensations and the uncomfortable ones, as well. Scan your body from the top of your head, noting any feelings on your scalp, going down toward your face, focusing on your eyes, down toward your nose, across to your ears, and down toward your mouth, lips, and farther down to your chin. Take in all the sensations and feelings graciously and tenderly. Be open to all that shows up and accept it for what it is. Just be with it.

From your chin, go down toward your collarbones, gently to your shoulders, sweeping down your chest, and notice as your lungs take in breaths. Inhale and exhale with rhythmic motion. Feel the air as it enters and exits your lungs.

Make your way toward your arms. Let your mind swoop down your arms slowly and meaningfully. Go farther down toward your fingers. Notice your hand and each and every finger. Notice their length as they expand outward.

Again, notice all feelings and sensations. Notice the comfortable sensations and the uncomfortable ones, as well. Take it all in graciously and tenderly. Be open to all that shows up and accept it for what it is. Just be with it.

Make your way to your pelvis and then down toward your thighs. In your mind's eye, think about energy cascading down your thighs in a circular motion, feeling each and every vibration. Go down to your legs. Feel their length and strength all the way through. Go down to your feet. How does each toe feel as you stretch it slowly and mindfully? Take it in graciously and tenderly. Be open to all that shows up and accept it for what it is. Just be with it fully.

Notice the wonder of your body and how it miraculously functions, how it generously serves you with openness, thoughtfulness, and kindness. Appreciate all that it has to offer you and feel deep gratitude that your body will continue to serve you always, all the days of your joyous and enriched life.

Congratulate yourself for your willingness and openness toward your journey.

Getting to the Finish Line

Sit comfortably and gently close your eyes.

Sit all the way back in your seat. Notice your feet touching the ground and the air that fills your lungs, with oxygen flowing in and your lungs being filled up. Notice how you exhale and how your body is relaxed, awaiting more air to fill your lungs. Without judgment, just notice it all from the top of your head all the way down to your feet. Notice every sensation, every feeling; notice if there's numbness, tingling, or any other sensation that may come up. Just notice it. Keep noticing it and then return to your breath. Your breath is reliable; it's there waiting for you.

You are entering a race—a race to go after what you want, what you believe in, what is meaningful to you, and what it is that you stand for. Imagine what that is for you. See that image clearly. Observe the image of you that you want so eagerly and passionately. Keep that image present in your mind, vividly and boldly.

It is so close, yet so far. You want to get rid of the barriers, the barricades, and the roadblocks. You want free access to what you want and to your vibrant image.

Imagine those barriers and how you would access what it is that you want. Look for an open space, a passageway, so you can make your way to it. Continue moving closer and realize that you are almost there, winning the race and getting all that you want.

Recognize that the image can and will become a reality if you push yourself a little harder—if you forge ahead and fight for what you want, need, and deserve. The finish line is near; it is just a foot away. It is yours if you grab for it, reach for it, and go for it.

You labor for it, and with all your will and might you manage to reach it. It is yours. You have access to it. No barriers, no barricades, and no roadblocks. It is all yours. You won the race. You crossed the finish line. You have what you wanted. You have what is meaningful to you.

It is no longer an image. It is a reality. You personally made it happen with your own strength and effort. You're incredible. Say to yourself, "My personal strength made it happen. I am resilient and I am persevering. I am incredible."

Congratulate yourself for your willingness and openness toward your journey.

The Sunset from the Mountaintop

Sit comfortably and gently close your eyes.

Notice how your body feels as you're sitting with an upright posture. Take a deep breath in. Notice how your lungs fill with air while you inhale and exhale. Continue to consciously breathe with full, deep breaths, noticing every inhalation and exhalation.

You are standing on a mountainside and observing the sunset. You notice an array of colors, the oranges and the yellows, blues, the purples and pinks. Your heart is feeling peaceful and at rest, and you watch as the sun sets gradually and steadily.

You notice what's all around you—the trees and branches and the valleys setting you apart from the other mountains. You notice your body and how it feels grounded. You notice the earth's hues. You notice the tans, the greens, the beiges, and the browns, the soothing colors that cover the earth. You notice the sun slowly descending. As it lowers gracefully, you watch with anticipation.

You notice the change in colors. They appear to slowly fade. You continue to feel your feet grounded on the floor and how your body is taking up space. You wait, you watch, you observe, and you stay connected to the moment.

The sun makes its final descent. You take one last look around you. Now you notice slopes and a river far in the distance. You notice the feeling of calmness in your body. You also notice how the hues change on the mountain and earth as the sun sets. You appreciate the impact and impression that the sun makes within you and the rest of the environment it shines over.

You continue to notice the stillness. The sun departs, making room for the night and all its glory. You continue to watch. You feel thankful for the present moment. You take a deep breath. A bigger, deeper breath than you ordinarily would. You notice how your lungs fill with air, and you feel grateful. You continue to consciously breathe with full, deep breaths. You notice how your body is reacting to that breath. It feels calmness and gratitude. You take that feeling with you as you quietly and slowly descend the mountain. You also take your openness and flexibility. You feel empowered to succeed and work hard and put all your efforts into being your best you and creating the life you want to live.

Congratulate yourself for your willingness and openness toward your journey.

You Hold the Power

Sit comfortably and gently close your eyes.

Be aware of your body and breathing. All parts of your body are wonderful, and all parts deserve recognition and appreciation. Just be with it all, as your body is always present. Your mind can ebb and flow toward the past and future, but your body will always be with you in the here and now, in the present moment.

Reflect on something that you feel went well for you today or yesterday. Think about what that was for you, whether it was acting kind to someone, doing well at something you were trying, or finishing something you were working on. Think about the pride you felt and the sense of appreciation and gratitude you had for yourself. Appreciate the beauty of that moment and the fact that you're able to notice yourself and all that you are. Notice that every day you are becoming stronger, more thoughtful, and more accomplished. You're always getting better with each moment that passes. You're an incredible person who holds so much value and love. At your core, you're warm, kind, and lovable.

You are the creator of your destiny. You have the ability to do or be anything that you set your mind's eye on. When you work hard at something, you strive and you accomplish. You always do, because you put all your energy into being who you want to be. Your mind is your only barrier. It sometimes tells you that you can't, that you won't, and that you don't know how to. You absolutely can. If you want to, you will, and if you don't know how to, you will learn how to. There aren't any barriers to doing what you want to do. You can do anything. You have the ability because you're powerful and wonderful. Embrace yourself, your abilities, your mind, your feelings, your actions, and who you fundamentally are.

Reflect on who you want to be. Have an image in your mind of something you would do or say to yourself or others. Have awareness of how that would feel in your body and in your heart. Identify the thoughts and feelings that go along with the image. Imagine that you're being congratulated for being who you want to be, that you feel proud of looking at and thinking of yourself. In your heart you feel joy, you feel peace, and you feel serenity and fulfillment. You are one with yourself because you are being who you want to be. You are the creator of your destiny.

As I walk with you throughout your journey, I am so proud of you. I am honored that you're taking me along on your journey. I enjoy being with you. You are such a gift to have around. I will continue to walk with you and will always support and nurture you as you go on your way. I am proud of all that you are.

Congratulate yourself for your willingness and openness toward your journey.

NOTES

INTRODUCTION

1 Ogden, C.L., Carroll, M.D., Fryar., C.D., and Flegal, K.M. (2015). "Prevalence of Obesity Among Adults and Youth: United States, 2011–2014." NCHS Data Brief, no 219. Hyattsville, MD: National Center for Health Statistics.

Ogden, C.L., Carroll, M.D., Kit, B.K., and Flegal, K.M. (2014). "Prevalence of Childhood and Adult Obesity in the United States, 2011–2012." *Journal of the American Medical Association (JAMA)*, 311(8), 806–14.

Ogden, C.L., Carroll, M.D., Kit, B.K., and Flegal, K.M. (2013). "Prevalence of Obesity Among Adults: United States, 2011–2012." NCHS Data Brief, no 131. Hyattsville, MD: National Center for Health Statistics.

Ogden, C.L., Carroll, M.D., Kit B.K., and Flegal, K.M. (2012). "Prevalence of Obesity in the United States, 2009–2010." NCHS Data Brief, no 82. Hyattsville, MD: National Center for Health Statistics.

Ogden, C., and Carroll, M. (2010). "Prevalence of Obesity Among Children and Adolescents: United States, Trends 1963–1965 Through 2007–2008." National Center for Health Statistics (NCHS) Health E-Stat.

2 Wang, D.D., Li, Y., Chiuve, S.E., Hu, F.B., Willett, W.C. (2015). "Improvements in US Diet Helped Reduce Disease Burden and Lower Premature Deaths, 1999–2012; Overall Diet Remains Poor." *Health Affairs*, 34(11), 1916–22.

3 Dalen, J., Brody, J.L., Staples, J.K, and Sedillo, D. (2015). "A Conceptual Framework for the Expansion of Behavioral Interventions for Youth Obesity: A Family-Based Mindful Eating Approach." *Childhood Obesity*, 11(5), 577–84.

4 Miller, W.R. (2013). *Motivational Interviewing: Helping People Change.* 3rd Edition. New York: Guilford Press.

Miller, W. (2009). "Motivational Interviewing: Facilitating Change Across Boundaries." YouTube video posted by columbiauniversity October 22, 2009. youtube.com/watch?v=6EeCirPyq2w

5 Mayo Clinic Staff. (2015). "Diseases and Conditions: Eating Disorders." mayoclinic.org, February 14, 2015.

6 Hayes, S.C. (2014). "The Mental Spider That Claims to Be Us." *Get Out of Your Mind* (blog), *Psychology Today*, February 19, 2012. Hayes notes he has changed the quote from Emo Philips from "brain" to "mind."

7 Kabat-Zinn, J. (1994). *Wherever You Go, There You Are: Mindfulness Meditation in Everyday Life*. New York: Hyperion. p. 4.

8 Davis, D.M., and Hayes, J.A. (2011). "What Are the Benefits of Mindfulness? A Practice Review of Psychotherapy-Related Research." *Psychotherapy*, 48(2), 198–208.

9 Brown, K.W., and Ryan, R.M. (2003). "The Benefits of Being Present: Mindfulness and Its Role in Psychological Well-being." *Journal of Personality and Social Psychology*, 84(4), 822–48.

Hölzel, B.K, Carmody, J., Vangel, M., et al. (2011). "Mindfulness Practice Leads to Increases in Regional Brain Gray Matter Density." *Psychiatry Research*, 191(1), 36–43.

Hutcherson, C., Seppala, E.M., and Gross, J.J., et al. (2008). "Loving-Kindness Meditation Increases Social Connectedness." *Emotion*, 8(5), 720–24.

Greeson, J.M. (2008). "Mindfulness Research Update: 2008." *Complementary Health Practice Review*, 14(1), 10–18.

Grossman, P., Tiefenthaler-Gilmer, U., Raysz, A., and Kesper, U. (2007). "Mindfulness Training as an Intervention for Fibromyalgia: Evidence of Postintervention and 3-Year Follow-up Benefits in Well-being." *Psychotherapy and Psychosomatics*, 76, 226–33.

Grossman, P., Niemann, L., Schmidt, S., and Walach, H. (2004). "Mindfulness-Based Stress Reduction and Health Benefits: A Meta-Analysis." *Journal of Psychosomatic Research*, 57(1), 35–43.

Kabat-Zinn, J. (1990). *Full Catastrophe Living: Using the Wisdom of Your Body and Mind to Face Stress, Pain, and Illness*. New York: Delacorte.

Kabat-Zinn, J., Lipworth, L., and Burney, R. (1985). "The Clinical Use of Mindfulness Meditation for the Self-Regulation of Chronic Pain." *Journal of Behavioral Medicine*, 8(2), 163–90.

Kristeller, J.L., and Hallett, C.B. (1999). "An Exploratory Study of a Meditation-Based Intervention for Binge Eating Disorder." *Journal of Health Psychology*, 4(3), 357–63.

Lazar, S.W., Kerr, C.E., Wasserman, R.H., et al. (2005). "Meditation Experience Is Associated with Increased Cortical Thickness." *NeuroReport*, 16(17), 1893–97.

Miller, J.J., Fletcher, K., and Kabat-Zinn, J. (1995). "Three-Year Follow-up and Clinical Implications of a Mindfulness-Based Stress Reduction Intervention in the Treatment of Anxiety Disorders." *General Hospital Psychiatry*, 17(3), 192–200.

Schreiner, I., and Malcolm, J.P. (2008). "The Benefits of Mindfulness Meditation: Changes in Emotional States of Depression, Anxiety, and Stress." *Behaviour Change*, 25(3), 156–68.

Shapiro, D., Cook, I.A., Davydov, D.M., et al. (2007). "Yoga as a Complementary Treatment of Depression: Effects of Traits and Moods on Treatment Outcome." *Evidence-Based Complementary and Alternative Medicine*, 4(4), 493–502.

Teasdale, J., Segal, Z.V., Williams, J.M., et al. (2000). "Prevention of Relapse/Recurrence in Major Depression by Mindfulness-Based Cognitive Therapy." *Journal of Counseling and Clinical Psychology*, 68(4), 615–23.

Zeidan, F., Johnson, S.K., Diamond, B.J., et al. (2010). "Mindfulness Meditation Improves Cognition: Evidence of Brief Mental Training." *Consciousness and Cognition*, 19(2), 597–605.

10 Pickert, K. (2014). "The Art of Being Mindful: Finding Peace in a Stressed-Out, Digitally Dependent Culture May Just Be a Matter of Thinking Differently." *Time*, February 3, 2014.

11 Black, D.S., Milam, J., and Sussman, S. (2009). "Sitting-Meditation Interventions Among Youth: A Review of Treatment Efficacy." *Pediatrics*, 124(3): e532–41.

Broderick, P.C., and Metz, S. (2009). "Learning to BREATHE: A Pilot Trial of a Mindfulness Curriculum for Adolescents." *Advances in Social Mental Health Promotion*, 2(1), 35–46.

Burke, C.A. (2009). "Mindfulness-Based Approaches with Children and Adolescents: A Preliminary Review of Current Research in an Emergent Field." *Journal of Child and Family Studies*, published online June 27, 2009.

Greenberg, M.T., and Harris, A.R. (2011). "Nurturing Mindfulness in Children and Youth: Current State of Research." *Child Development Perspectives*, published online October 31, 2011.

Harrison, L.J., Manocha, R., and Rubia, K. (2004). "Sahaja Yoga Meditation as a Family Treatment Programme with Attention Deficit-Hyperactivity Disorder." *Clinical Child Psychology and Psychiatry*, 9(4), 479–97.

Meiklejohn, J., Phillips, C., Freedman, M.L., et al. (2012). "Integrating Mindfulness Training into K–12 Education: Fostering the Resilience of Teachers and Students." *Mindfulness*, March 14, 2012.

Rosaen, C., and Benn, R. (2006). "The Experience of Transcendental Meditation in Middle School Students: A Qualitative Report." *Explore*, 2(5), 422–25.

Sibinga, E.M., Kerrigan, D., Stewart, M., et al. (2011). "Mindfulness-Based Stress Reduction for Urban Youth." *Journal of Alternative and Complementary Medicine*, 17(3), 213–18.

Singh, N., Lancioni, G.E., Singh Joy, S.E., et al. (2007). "Adolescents with Conduct Disorder Can Be Mindful of Their Aggressive Behavior." *Journal of Emotional and Behavioral Disorders*, 15(1), 56–63.

Wall, R.B. (2005). "Tai Chi and Mindfulness-Based Stress Reduction in a Boston Public Middle School." *Journal of Pediatric Health Care*, 19(4), 230–37.

12 Chodkowski, B.A., Cowan, R.L., and Niswender, K.D. (2016). "Imbalance in Resting State Functional Connectivity Is Associated with Eating Behavior and Adiposity in Children." Heliyon, 2, published online January 21, 2016.

13 Pickert, K. "The Art of Being Mindful."

14 Hooker, K.E., and Fodor, I.E. (2008). "Teaching Mindfulness to Children." *Gestalt Review*, 12(1), 75–91.

15 Stoddard, J.A., and Afari, N. (2014). *The Big Book of ACT Metaphors: A Practitioner's Guide to Experiential Exercises and Metaphors in Acceptance and Commitment Therapy.* Oakland, CA: New Harbinger Publications.

16 Mayo Clinic (2013). "Mindfulness: Learning to Live in the Moment." Special Report, Supplement to *Mayo Clinic Health Letter,* October 2013.

17 Wansink, B., and Sobal, J. (2007). "Mindless Eating: The 200 Daily Food Decisions We Overlook." *Environment and Behavior,* 39(1), 106–23.

18 Westrup, D. (2014). *Advanced Acceptance and Commitment Therapy: The Experienced Practitioner's Guide to Optimizing Delivery.* Oakland, CA: New Harbinger Publications.

19 Hayes, S.C., Strosahl, K.D., and Wilson, K.G. (1999). *Acceptance and Commitment Therapy: An Experiential Approach to Behavior Change.* New York: Guilford Press.

Titchener, E.B. (1916). *A Text-Book of Psychology.* New York: Macmillian. (See the *Milk, Milk, Milk* exercises.)

CHAPTER 2

20 Harris, R. (2008). *The Happiness Trap: How to Stop Struggling and Start Living.* Boston: Shambhala Publications.

21 Stoddard, J.A., and Niloofar, A. (2014). *The Big Book of ACT Metaphors: A Practitioner's Guide to Experiential Exercises and Metaphors in Acceptance and Commitment Therapy.* Oakland, CA: New Harbinger Publications.

22 Pearson, A.N., Heffner, M., and Follette, V.M. (2010). *Acceptance and Commitment Therapy for Body Image Dissatisfaction: A Practitioner's Guide to Using Mindfulness, Acceptance, and Values-Based Behavior Change Strategies.* Oakland, CA: New Harbinger Publications.

23 Stoddard and Niloofar, *The Big Book of ACT Metaphors.*

24 Hayes, S.C., Strosahl, K.D, and Wilson, K.G. (2012). *Acceptance and Commitment Therapy: The Process and Practice of Mindful Change* (2nd ed.). New York: Guilford Press.

25 Lillis, J., Dahl, J., and Weineland, S.M. (2014). *The Diet Trap: Feed Your Psychological Needs and End the Weight Loss Struggle Using Acceptance and Commitment Therapy.* Oakland, CA: New Harbinger Publications.

26 Pearson, Heffner, and Follette, *Acceptance and Commitment Therapy for Body Image Dissatisfaction.*

27 Ciarrochi, J., Bailey, A., and Harris, R. (2014). *The Weight Escape: How to Stop Dieting and Start Living: Lose Weight and Reshape Your Life Using the Mindfulness-Based Methods of ACT: Acceptance and Commitment Therapy.* Boston: Shambhala Publications. p. 20.

28 Ciarrochi, J.V., Hayes, L., and Bailey, A. (2012). *Get Out of Your Mind and Into Your Life for Teens: A Guide to Living an Extraordinary Life.* Oakland, CA: New Harbinger Publications.

Dahl, J.C., Plumb, J.C., Stewart, I., and Lundgren, T. (2009). *The Art and Science of Valuing in Psychotherapy: Helping Clients Discover, Explore, and Commit to Valued Action Using Acceptance and Commitment Therapy.* Oakland, CA: New Harbinger Publications.

29 Westrup, D. (2014). *Advanced Acceptance and Commitment Therapy: The Experienced Practitioner's Guide to Optimizing Delivery*. Oakland, CA: New Harbinger Publications.

30 Ciarrochi, Bailey, and Harris, *The Weight Escape: How to Stop Dieting and Start Living*.

CHAPTER 3

31 Beck, J.S. (2011). *Cognitive Behavior Therapy: Basics and Beyond* (2nd ed.). New York: Guilford Press.

32 Beck, J. (2007). *The Beck Diet Solution: Train Your Brain to Think Like a Thin Person*. Birmingham, AL: Oxmoor House.

33 Ibid.

34 McQuillian, S. (2004). *Psychology Today: Breaking the Bonds of Food Addiction*. New York: Alpha.

35 Zelman, K.M. (2015). "Am I Really Hungry? 5 Ways to Get in Touch with Your Appetite." webmd.com, January 22, 2015.

36 Satter, Ellyn. (1987). *How to Get Your Kids to Eat: But Not Too Much*. Boulder, CO: Bull Publishing.

Satter, Ellyn. (2011). *Your Child's Weight: Helping Without Harming*. Madison, WI: Kelcy Press.

37 Adapted from Beck, J.S. (2008). *The Beck Diet Solution: Train Your Brain to Think Like a Thin Person*. Birmingham, AL: Oxmoor House.

38 Taitz, J.L. (2012). *End Emotional Eating: Using Dialectical Behavior Therapy Skills to Cope with Difficult Emotions and Develop a Healthy Relationship with Food*. Oakland, CA: New Harbinger Publications.

39 Ibid.

40 Mayo Clinic (2013). *Mindfulness: Learning to Live in the Moment*. Special Report, Supplement to *Mayo Clinic Health Letter*, October 2013. p. 5.

41 Wansink, B., Cheney, M.M., and Chan, N. (2003). "Exploring Comfort Food Preferences Across Age and Gender." *Physiology and Behavior*, 79(4–5), 739–47.

Wansink, B., and Sangerman, C. (2000). "Engineering Comfort Foods." *American Demographics*, July 2000, 66–67.

42 Jakubczak, J. "Emotional Eating: Feeding Your Feelings." webmd.com.

43 Scaglioni, S., Salvioni, M., and Galimberti, C. (2008). "Influence of Parental Attitudes in the Development of Children Eating Behaviour." *British Journal of Nutrition*, 99, S22–25.

44 Tribole, E., and Resch, E. (2012). *Intuitive Eating* (3rd ed.). New York: St. Martin's Griffin.

45 May, M. (2011). "Eat What You Love, Love What You Eat: How to Break Your Eat-Repent-Repeat Cycle." Austin, TX: Greenleaf Book Group Press.

46 Zelman, K. (2012). "Portion Control and Size Guide." webmd.com, September 27, 2012. Adapted.

47 MacDonald, A. (2010). "Why Eating Slowly May Help You Feel Full Faster." *Harvard Health Publications. Harvard Medical School. Harvard Health Blog.* October 19, 2010. health.harvard.edu.

48 Rolls, B.J. (2014). "What Is the Role of Portion Control in Weight Management?" *International Journal of Obesity*, 38, S1–8.

49 Hayman, M. (2014). "Food Addiction: Could It Explain Why 70 Percent of Americans Are Fat?" *Dr. Mark Hyman* (blog) and *Huffington Post.* October 16, 2010. drhyman.com and huffingtonpost.com.

50 Snoek, H.M., Engels, R., Janssens, J.M., and van Strien, T. (2007). "Parental Behavior and Adolescents' Emotional Eating." *Appetite*, 49(1), 223–30.

CHAPTER 4

51 Beck, A.T. (1963). "Thinking and Depression: Idiosyncratic Content and Cognitive Distortions." *Archives of General Psychiatry*, 9, 324–33.

Beck, A.T. (1964). "Thinking and Depression: Theory and Therapy." *Archives of General Psychiatry*, 10, 561–71.

52 Adapted from Beck, J.S. (2008). *The Beck Diet Solution: Train Your Brain to Think Like a Thin Person.* Birmingham, AL: Oxmoor House.

53 Ibid.

CHAPTER 5

54 Ahrendt, A.D., Kattelmann, K.K., Rector, T.S., and Maddox, D.A. (2013). "The Effectiveness of Telemedicine for Weight Management in the MOVE! Program." *Journal of Rural Health*, 30(1), 113–19.

Donaldson, E.L., Fallows, S., and Morris, M. (2014). "A Text Message Based Weight Management Intervention for Overweight Adults." *Journal of Human Nutrition and Dietetics*, 27(2), 90–97.

Entwistle, P.A., Webb, R.J, Abayomi, J.C., et al. (2014). "Unconscious Agendas in the Etiology of Refractory Obesity and the Role of Hypnosis in Their Identification and Resolution: A New Paradigm for Weight-Management Programs or a Paradigm Revisited?" *International Journal of Clinical and Experimental Hypnosis*, 62(3), 330–59.

55 Marketdata Enterprises. (2014). *The U.S. Weight Loss Market: 2014 Status Report and Forecast.* February 1, 2014. marketresearch.com/Marketdata-Enterprises-Inc-v416/Weight-Loss-Status-Forecast-8016030.

56 MacMillian, A. (2011). "After Dieting, Hormone Changes May Fuel Weight Regain." cnn.com. October 26, 2011.

57 Mann, T., Tomiyama, A.J., Westling, E., et al. (2007). "Medicare's Search for Effective Obesity Treatments: Diets Are Not the Answer." *American Psychologist*, 62(3), 220–33.

58 Zeevi, D., Korem, T., Zmora, N., et al., (2015). "Personalized Nutrition by Prediction of Glycemic Responses." *Cell*, 163(5), 1079–94.

59 Pietiläinen, K.H., Saarni, S.E., Kaprio J., and Rissanen, A. (2012). "Does Dieting Make You Fat? A Twin Study." *International Journal of Obesity*, 36(3), 456–64.

60 Field, A.E., Austin, S.B., Taylor, C.B., et al. (2003). "Relation Between Dieting and Weight Change Among Preadolescents and Adolescents." *Pediatrics*, 112(4), 900–6.

61 Neumark-Sztainer, D., Wall, M., Guo, J., et al. (2006). "Obesity, Disordered Eating, and Eating Disorders in a Longitudinal Study of Adolescents: How Do Dieters Fare 5 Years Later?" *Journal of the American Dietetic Association*, 106(4), 559–68.

62 Haines, J., and Neumark-Sztainer, D. (2006). "Prevention of Obesity and Eating Disorders: A Consideration of Shared Risk Factors." *Health Education Research*, 21(6), 770–82.

Patton, G.C., Selzer, R., Coffey, C., et al. (1999). "Onset of Adolescent Eating Disorders: Population Based Cohort Study over 3 Years." *British Medical Journal*, 318, 765–68.

63 DiSalvo, D. (2014). "Not by Willpower Alone: Willpower Is Essential Fuel, But It Needs Help to Move Us Forward." *Psychology Today*. May/June 2014.

64 Phillippa, L., van Jaarsveld, C.H.M., Potts, H.W.W., and Wardle, J. (2010). "How Are Habits Formed: Modelling Habit Formation in the Real World." *European Journal of Social Psychology*, 40(6), 998–1009.

CHAPTER 6

65 Svensson, V., Jacobsson, J.A., Fredriksson, R, et al. (2011). "Associations Between Severity of Obesity in Childhood and Adolescence, Obesity Onset and Parental BMI: A Longitudinal Cohort Study." *International Journal of Obesity*, 35(1), 46–52.

66 Beck, J.S. (2011). *Cognitive Behavior Therapy: Basics and Beyond* (2nd ed.). New York: Guilford Press.

Dobson, K.S. (2012). *Cognitive Therapy*. Washington, DC: APA Books.

67 Ormrod, J.E. (2006). *Educational Psychology: Developing Learners* (5th ed.), Upper Saddle River, NJ: Pearson/Merrill Prentice Hall.

68 Bandura, A. (1994). "Self-Efficacy." In V.S. Ramachaudran (Ed.), *Encyclopedia of Human Behavior*, Vol. 4, New York: Academic Press, pp. 71–81.

69 Beck, A.T. (1976). *Cognitive Therapy and the Emotional Disorders*. New York: Meridian.

70 Luszczynska, A., and Schwarzer, R. (2005). "Social Cognitive Theory." In M. Conner and P. Norman (Eds.), *Predicting Health Behaviour* (2nd ed. Rev.), Buckingham, England: Open University Press, pp. 127–69.

71 Van Beek, M., Sanford Children's Clinic, Sioux Falls, SD, quoted in Barker, J. (2012). "Keeping a Kid's Weight in Perspective." webmd.com. January 11, 2012.

72 Dalen, J., Brody, J.L., Staples, J.K, and Sedillo, D. (2015). "A Conceptual Framework for the Expansion of Behavioral Interventions for Youth Obesity: A Family-Based Mindful Eating Approach." *Childhood Obesity*, 11(5), 577–84.

Epstein, L.H., Paluch, R.A., Roemmich, J.N., and Beecher, M.D. (2007). "Family-Based Obesity Treatment, Then and Now: Twenty-Five Years of Pediatric Obesity Treatment." *Health Psychology*, 26(4), 381–91.

Hampl, S., Odar Stough, C., Poppert Cordts, K., et al. (2016). "Effectiveness of a Hospital-Based Multidisciplinary Pediatric Weight Management Program: Two-Year Outcomes of PHIT Kids." *Childhood Obesity*, 12(1), 20-5.

73 Ervin, R.B., Kit, B.K., Carroll, M.D., and Ogden, C.L. (2012). "Consumption of Added Sugar Among U.S. Children and Adolescents, 2005–2008." NCHS Data Brief, no 87. Hyattsville, MD: National Center for Health Statistics.

74 CASA. (2010). *The Importance of Family Dinners VI*. National Center on Addiction and Substance Abuse, Columbia University. casacolumbia.org.

Eisenberg, M.E., Neumark-Sztainer, D., Fulkerson, J.A., and Story, M. (2008). "Family Meals and Substance Use: Is There a Long-term Protective Association?" *Journal of Adolescent Health*, 43, 151–56.

Eisenberg, M.E., Olson, R.E., Neumark-Sztainer, D., et al. (2004). "Correlations Between Family Meals and Psychosocial Well-being Among Adolescents." *Archives of Pediatric and Adolescent Medicine*, 158, 792–96.

Fiese, B.H., Foley, K.P., and Spagnola, M. (2006). "Routine and Ritual Elements in Family Mealtimes: Contexts for Child Well-being and Family Identity." *New Directions for Child and Adolescent Development*, 111, 67–89.

Fiese, B.H., and Hammons, A.J. (2011). "Is Frequency of Shared Family Meals Related to the Nutritional Health of Children and Adolescents?" *Journal of the American Academy of Pediatrics*, 127, 1565–74.

Fisher, L.B., Miles, I.W., Austin, S.B., et al. (2007). "Predictors of Initiation of Alcohol Use Among US Adolescents: Findings from a Prospective Cohort Study." *Archives of Pediatrics and Adolescent Medicine*, 161, 959–66.

Fulkerson, J.A., Kubik, M.Y., Story, M., et al. (2009). "Are There Nutritional and Other Benefits Associated with Family Meals Among At-Risk Youth?" *Journal of Adolescent Health*, 45, 389–95.

Fulkerson, J.A., Story, M., Mellin, A., et al. (2006). "Family Dinner Meal Frequency and Adolescent Development: Relationships with Developmental Assets and High-Risk Behaviors." *Journal of Adolescent Health*, 39, 337–45.

Griffin, K.W., Botvin, G.J., Scheier, L.M., et al. (2000). "Parenting Practices as Predictors of Substance Use, Delinquency, and Aggression Among Urban Minority Youth: Moderating Effects of Family Structure and Gender." *Psychology of Addictive Behaviors*, 14, 17–84.

Musick, K., and Meier, A. (2012). "Assessing Causality and Persistence in Associations Between Family Dinners and Adolescent Well-being." *Journal of Marriage and Family*, 74(3), 476–93.

Neumark-Sztainer, D., Hannan, P.J., Story, M., et al. (2003). "Family Meal Patterns: Associations with Sociodemographic Characteristics and Improved Dietary Intake Among Adolescents." *Journal of the American Dietetic Association*, 103, 317–22.

Sen, B. (2010). "The Relationship Between Frequency of Family Diner and Adolescent Problem Behaviors After Adjusting for Other Family Characteristics." *Journal of Adolescence*, 33, 187–96.

Taveras, E.M., Rifas-Shiman, S.L., Berkey, C.S., et al. (2005). "Family Dinner and Adolescent Overweight." *Obesity Research*, 13, 900–6.

Videon, T.M., and Manning, C.K. (2003). "Influences on Adolescent Eating Patterns: The Importance of Family Meals." *Journal of Adolescent Health*, 32, 365–73.

75 AAP Council on Communications and Media (2011). "Media Use by Children Younger Than 2 Years." *Pediatrics*, 128(5), 1040–45.

Page, A.S., Cooper, A.R., Griew, P., and Jago, R. (2010). "Children's Screen Viewing Is Related to Psychological Difficulties Irrespective of Physical Activity." *Pediatrics*, 126(5), 1011–17.

Wijga, A.H., Scholtens, S., Bemelmans, W.J.E., et al. (2010). "Diet, Screen Time, Physical Activity, and Childhood Overweight in the General Population and in High Risk Subgroups: Prospective Analyses in the PIAMA Birth Cohort." *Journal of Obesity*, 2010, Article ID 423296. hindawi.com.

Landhuis, E.C., Poulton, R., Welch, D., and Hancox R.J. (2008). "Programming Obesity and Poor Fitness: The Long-term Impact of Childhood Television." *Obesity*, 16(6), 1457–59.

Jago, R., Baranowski, T., Baranowski, J.C., et al. (2005). "BMI from 3–6 Years of Age Is Predicted by TV Viewing and Physical Activity, Not Diet." *International Journal of Obesity*, 29(6), 557–64.

Weicha, J.L., Peterson, K.E., Ludwig, D.S., et al. (2006). "When Children Eat What They Watch: Impact of Television Viewing on Dietary Intake in Youth." *Archives of Pediatric and Adolescent Medicine*, 60, 436–42. archpedi.jamanetwork.com.

Harrison, K., Liechty, J.M., and the Strong Kids Program (2011). "US Preschoolers' Media Exposure and Dietary Habits: The Primacy of Television and the Limits of Parental Mediation." *Journal of Children and Media*, 6(1), 18–36.

Tavaras, E.M., Sandora, T.J., Shih, M.C., et al. (2006). "The Association of Television and Video Viewing with Fast Food Intake by Preschool-Age Children." *Obesity*, 14, 2034–41.

Adachi-Mejia, A.M., Longacre, M.R., Gibson. J.J., et al. (2007). "Children with a TV in Bedroom at Higher Risk for Being Overweight." *International Journal of Obesity*, 31(4), 644–51.

Taveras, E.M., Hohman, K.H., Price, S., et al. (2009). "Televisions in the Bedrooms of Racial/Ethnic Minority Children: How Did They Get There and How Do We Get Them Out?" *Clinical Pediatrics*, 48(7), 715–19.

Chaput, J.P., Visby, T., Nyby, S., et al. (2011). "Video Game Playing Increases Food Intake in Adolescents: A Randomized Crossover Study." *American Journal of Clinical Nutrition*, 93(6), 1196–203.

Baranowski, T., Abdelsamad, D., Baranowski, J., et al. (2012). "Impact of an Active Video Game on Healthy Children's Physical Activity." *Pediatrics*, 129(3), e636–42. pediatrics.aappublications.org.

Epstein, L.H., Roemmich, J.N., Robinson, J.L., et al. (2008). "A Randomized Trial of the Effects of Reducting Television Viewing and Computer Use on Body Mass Index in Young Children." *Archives of Pediatric and Adolescent Medicine*, 162(3), 239–45. archpedi.jamanetwork.com.

76 AAP Council on Communications and Media (2013). "Children, Adolescents, and the Media," *Pediatrics*, October 28, 2013. pediatrics.aappublications.org.

77 National Sleep Foundation. "Children and Sleep." sleepfoundation.org/sleep-topics/children-and-sleep.

78 Patel, S.R., and Hu, F.B. (2008). "Short Sleep Duration and Weight Gain: A Systematic Review." *Obesity*, 16, 643–53.

Reilly, J.J., Armstrong, J., Dorosty, A.R., et al. (2005). "Early Life Risk Factors for Obesity in Childhood: Cohort Study." *BMJ*, 330, 1357.

Gillman, M.W., Rifas-Shiman, S.L., Kleinman, K., et al. (2008). "Developmental Origins of Childhood Overweight: Potential Public Health Impact." *Obesity*, 16, 1651–56.

Taveras, E.M., Rifas-Shiman, S.L., Oken, E., et al. (2008). "Short Sleep Duration in Infancy and Risk of Childhood Overweight." *Archives of Pediatrics and Adolescent Medicine*, 162, 305–11.

Bell, J.F., and Zimmerman, F.J. (2010). "Shortened Nighttime Sleep Duration in Early Life and Subsequent Childhood Obesity." *Archives of Pediatrics and Adolescent Medicine*, 164, 840–45.

Landhuis, C.E., Poulton, R., Welch, D., and Hancox, R.J. (2008). "Childhood Sleep Time and Long-term Risk for Obesity: A 32-Year Prospective Birth Cohort Study." *Pediatrics*, 122, 955–60.

CHAPTER 7

79 Schwartz, M.B., and Puhl, R. (2003). "Childhood Obesity: A Societal Problem to Solve." *Obesity Reviews*, 4(1), 57–71.

80 Edmunds, L.D. (2005). "Parents' Perceptions of Health Professionals' Responses When Seeking Help for Their Overweight Children." *Family Practice*, 22, 287–92.

Pierce, J.W., and Wardle, J. (1997). "Cause and Effect Beliefs and Self-esteem of Overweight Children." *Journal of Child Psychology and Psychiatry*, 38, 645–50.

81 Turner, K.M., Salisbury, C., and Shield, J.P.H. (2011). "Parents' Views and Experiences of Childhood Obesity Management in Primary Care: A Qualitative Study." *Family Practice*, 29(4), 476–81.

82 Puhl, R.M., and Latner, J.D. (2007) "Stigma, Obesity, and the Health of the Nation's Children." *Psychological Bulletin*, 133(4), 557–80.

83 Davidson, K.K., and Birch, L.L. (2004). "Predictors of Fat Stereotypes Among 9-Year-Old Girls and Their Parents." *Obesity Research*, 12, 86–94.

84 Singh, A.S., Mulder, C., Twisk, J.W., et al. (2008). "Tracking of Childhood Overweight into Adulthood: A Systematic Review of the Literature." *Obesity Reviews*, 9, 474–88.

85 Dietz, W.H. (1998). "Childhood Weight Affects Adult Morbidity and Mortality." *Journal of Nutrition*, 128(2), 411S–14S.

Ebbeling, C.B., Pawlak, D.B., and Ludwig, D.S. (2002). "Childhood Obesity: Public-Health Crisis, Common Sense Cure." *Lancet*, 360, 473–82.

Janssen, I., Katzmarzyk, P.T., Srinivasan, S.R., et al. (2005). "Utility of Childhood BMI in the Prediction of Adulthood Disease: Comparison of National and International References." *Obesity Research*, 13(6), 1106–15.

Kuczmarski, R.J., Ogden, C.L., Grummer-Strawn, L.M., et al. (2000). "CDC Growth Charts: United States." *Advance Data*, 314. Hyattsville, MD: National Center for Health Statistics.

Ogden, C., and Carroll, M. (2012). "Prevalence of Obesity Among Children and Adolescents: United States, Trends 1963–1965 Through 2007–2008." National Center for Health Statistics (NCHS) Health E-Stat.

Ogden, C.L., Carroll, M.D., Kit, B.K., and Flegal, K.M. (2012). "Prevalence of Obesity in the United States, 2009–2010." NCHS Data Brief, no 82. Hyattsville, MD: National Center for Health Statistics.

Ogden, C.L., Carroll, M.D., Kit, B.K., and Flegal, K.M. (2013). "Prevalence of Obesity Among Adults: United States, 2011–2012." NCHS Data Brief, no 131. Hyattsville, MD: National Center for Health Statistics.

Troiano, R.P., and Flegal, K.M. (1998). "Overweight Children and Adolescents: Description, Epidemiology, and Demographics." *Pediatrics*, 101(3), 497–504.

86 Berge, J.M., MacLehose, R., Loth, K.A., et al. (2013). "Parent Conversations About Healthful Eating and Weight." *JAMA Pediatrics*, 167(8), 746–53.

87 Ibid.

88 Dell'Antonia, K.J. (2012). "When Teasing Is Loving, and When It's Not." *Motherlode* (blog), *The New York Times*, June 6, 2012.

89 Kluck, A.S. (2010). "Family Influence on Disordered Eating: The Role of Body Image Dissatisfaction." *Body Image*, 7(1), 8–14.

90 Eisenberg, M.E., Berge, J.M., Fulkerson, J.A., and Neumark-Sztainer, D. (2011). "Weight Comments by Family and Significant Others in Young Adulthood." *Body Image*, 8(1), 12–19.

91 Thompson, J.K, Heinberg, L.J., Albate, M.N., and Tantleff-Dunn, S. (1999). "Appearance-Related Feedback." In *Exacting Beauty: Theory, Assessment, and Treatment of Body Image Disturbance*, Washington, DC: APA Books, pp. 151–74.

92 Puhl and Latner, "Stigma, Obesity, and the Health of the Nation's Children."

93 Cash, T.F. (1995). "Developmental Teasing About Physical Appearance: Retrospective Descriptions and Relationships with Body Image." *Social Behavior and Personality*, 23(2), 123–30.

Rieves, L., and Cash, T.F., (1996). "Social Developmental Factors and Women's Body-Image Attitudes." *Journal of Social Behavior and Personality*, 2(1), 63–78.

94 Neumark-Sztainer, D.R., Wall, M.M., Haines, J.I., et al. (2007). "Shared Risk and Protective Factors for Overweight and Disordered Eating in Adolescents." *American Journal of Preventive Medicine*, 33(5), 359–69, E3.

95 Grodsten, F., Levine, R., Troy, L., et al. (1996). "Three-Year Follow-up of Participants in a Commercial Weight Loss Program: Can You Keep It Off?" *Archives of Internal Medicine*, 156(12), 1302.

Neumark-Sztainer, D., Haines, J., Wall, M., and Eisenberg, M.E. (2007). "Why Does Dieting Predict Weight Gain in Adolescents? Findings from Project EAT-II: A 5-Year Longitudinal Study." *Journal of the American Dietetic Association*, 107(3), 448–55.

96 Neumark-Sztainer, D. (2005). *"I'm, Like, SO Fat!": Helping Your Teen Make Healthy Choices About Eating and Exercise in a Weight-Obsessed World.* New York: Guilford Press.

97 Lindsay, A.C., Sussner, K.M., Kim, J., and Gortmaker, S. (2006). "The Role of Parents in Preventing Childhood Obesity." *The Future of Children*, 16(1), 169–86.

98 Aronne, L.J., Nelinson, D.S., and Lillo, J.L. (2009). "Obesity as a Disease State: A New Paradigm for Diagnosis and Treatment." *Clinic Cornerstone*, 9(4), 9–25, discussion 26–29.

99 Bray, G.A., Smith, S.R., de Jonge, L., et al. (2012). "Effect of Dietary Protein Content on Weight Gain, Energy Expenditure, and Body Composition During Overeating: A Randomized Control Trial." *JAMA*, 307(1), 47–55.

Hyman, M. (2012). *The Blood Sugar Solution: The UltraHealthy Program for Losing Weight, Preventing Disease, and Feeling Great Now!* New York: Little, Brown.

Li, Z., and Heber, D. (2012). "Overeating and Overweight: Extra Calories Increase Fat Mass While Protein Increases Lean Mass." *JAMA*, 307(1), 86–87.

100 Thaler, J.P., Yi, C.X., Schur, E.A., et al. (2012). "Obesity Is Associated with Hypothalamic Injury in Rodents and Humans." *Journal of Clinical Investigation*, 122(1), 153–62.

101 Gearhardt, A.N., Grilo, C.M., DiLeone, R.J., et al. (2011). "Can Food Be Addictive: Public Health and Policy Implications." *Addiction*, 106(7), 1208–12.

102 Volkow, N.D., Wang, G.J., Fowler, J.S., et al. (2002). "'Nonhedonic' Food Motivation in Humans Involves Dopamine in the Dorsal Striatum Methylphenidate Amplifies This Effect." *Synapse*, 44(3), 175–80.

103 Lenoir, M., Serre, F., Cantin, L., and Ahmed, S.H. (2007). "Intense Sweetness Surpasses Cocaine Reward." *PLOS ONE*, 2(8), e698.

Ahmed, S.H., Guillem, K., and Vandaele, Y. (2013). "Sugar Addiction: Pushing the Drug-Sugar Analogy to the Limit." *Current Opinion in Clinical Nutrition and Metabolic Care*, 16(4), 434–39.

Madsen, H.B., and Ahmed, S.H. (2014). "Drug Versus Sweet Reward: Greater Attraction to and Preference for Sweet Versus Drug Cues." *Addiction Biology*, published online March 7, 2014.

104 Ervin, R.B., Kit, B.K., Carroll, M.D., and Ogden, C.L. (2012). "Consumption of Added Sugar Among U.S. Children and Adolescents, 2005–2008." NCHS Data Brief, no 87. Hyattsville, MD: National Center for Health Statistics.

CHAPTER 8

105 Sales, J.M., and Irwin, C.E. (2013). "A Biopsychosocial Perspective of Adolescent Health and Disease." In W.T. O'Donohue, L.T. Benuto, and L. Woodward Tolle (Eds.), *Handbook of Adolescent Health Psychology*, New York: Springer Science+Business Media.

Hatala, A.R. (2012). "The Status of the 'Biopsychosocial' Model in Health Psychology: Towards an Integrated Approach and a Critique of Cultural Conceptions." *Open Journal of Medical Psychology*, 1(4), 51–62.

106 Erikson, E.H. (1980). *Identity and the Life Cycle.* New York: W.W. Norton. (Based on his Psychosocial Stages of Development)

107 Centers for Disease Control and Prevention. (2014). "Youth Risk Behavior Surveillance – United States, 2013." *Morbidity and Mortality Weekly Report (MMWR)*, 63(4).

108 Ogden C.L., Carroll, M.D., Kit, B.K., and Flegal, K.M. (2014). "Prevalence of Childhood and Adult Obesity in the United States, 2011–2012." *JAMA*, 311(8), 806–14.

109 Harris, J.L., Schwartz, M.B., LoDolce, M., et al. (2014). *Sugary Drink FACTS 2014: Food Advertising to Children and Teens Score.* Yale Rudd Center for Food Policy and Obesity. sugarydrinkfacts.org/resources/SugaryDrinkFACTS_Report.pdf.

110 Levine, M. (1998). "Prevention of Eating Problems with Elementary Children." *USA Today*, July 1998.

111 Puhl, R.M., and Kyle, T.K. (2014). "Pervasive Bias: An Obstacle to Obesity Solutions." Commentary. Washington, DC: Institute of Medicine.

Puhl, R.M., Andreyeva, T., and Brownell, K.D. (2008). "Perceptions of Weight Discrimination: Prevalence and Comparison to Race and Gender Discrimination in America." *International Journal of Obesity*, 32, 992–1000.

Andreyeva, T., Puhl, R.M., and Brownell, K.D. (2008). "Changes in Perceived Weight Discrimination Among Americans, 1995–1996 Through 2004–2006." *Obesity Journal*, 16(5), 1129–34.

112 Puhl, R.M., Luedicke, J., and Heuer, C. (2011). "Weight-Based Victimization Toward Overweight Adolescents: Observations and Reactions of Peers." *Journal of School Health*, 81, 696–703.

113 Bradshaw, C.P., Waasdorp, T.E., O'Brennan, L.M., and Gulemetova, M. (2011). *Findings from the National Education Association's Nationwide Study of Bullying: Teachers' and Education Professionals' Perspectives.* National Education Association. nea.org.

Puhl, R.M., Luedicke, J., and DePierre, J.A. (2013). "Parental Concerns About Weight-Based Victimization in Youth." *Childhood Obesity*, 9(6), 540–48.

114 Puhl, R.M., Peterson, J.L., and Luedicke J. (2013). "Weight-Based Victimization: Bullying Experiences of Weight loss Treatment–Seeking Youth." *Pediatrics*, 131(1), e1–9.

115 Neumark-Sztainer, D., Story, M., and Harris, T. (1999). "Beliefs and Attitudes About Obesity Among Teachers and School Health Care Providers Working with Adolescents." *Journal of Nutrition Education*, 31(1), 3–9.

116 O'Brian, K.S., Hunter, J.A., and Banks, M. (2007). "Implicit Anti-Fat Bias in Physical Educators: Physical Attributes, Ideology and Socialization." *International Journal of Obesity*, 31, 308–14.

117 Hatzenbuehler, M.L., Keyes, K.M., and Hasin, D.S. (2009). "Associations Between Perceived Weight Discrimination and the Prevalence of Psychiatric Disorders in the General Population." *Obesity*, 17(11), 2033–39.

118 Puhl, R.M., and Latner, J.D. (2007). "Stigma, Obesity, and the Health of the Nation's Children." *Psychological Bulletin*, 133(4), 557–80.

Eisenberg, M.E., Neumark-Sztainer, D., and Story, M. (2003). "Associations of Weight-Based Teasing and Emotional Well-being Among Adolescents." *Archives of Pediatrics and Adolescent Medicine*, 157(8), 733–38.

119 Quick, V.M., McWilliams, R., and Byrd-Bredbenner, C. (2013). "Fatty, Fatty, Two-by-Four: Weight-Teasing History and Disturbed Eating in Young Adult Women." *American Journal of Public Health*, 103(3), 508–15.

Libbey, H.P, Story, M.T., Neumark-Sztainer, D.R., and Boutelle, K.N. (2008). "Teasing, Disordered Eating Behaviors, and Psychological Morbidities Among Overweight Adolescents." *Obesity*, 16(2), S24–29.

120 Sutin, A.R., and Terracciano, A. (2013). "Perceived Weight Discrimination and Obesity." *PLOS ONE*. July 24, 2013.

121 Paul, R.M., and Luedicke, J. (2011). Weight-Based Victimization Among Adolescents in the School Setting: Emotional Reactions and Coping Behaviors." *Journal of Youth and Adolescence*, 41(1), 27–40.

Krukowski, R.A., West, D.S., Perez, A.P., et al. (2009). "Overweight Children, Weight-Based Teasing and Academic Performance." *International Journal of Pediatric Obesity*, 4(4), 274–80.

122 Robinson, S. (2006). "Victimization of Obese Adolescents." *Journal of School Nursing*, 22(4), 201.

123 Puhl, R.M., Peterson, J.L., and Luedicke, J. (2012). "Strategies to Address Weight-Based Victimization: Youths' Preferred Support Interventions from Classmates, Teachers, and Parents." *Journal of Youth and Adolescence*, 42(3), 315–27.

124 Puhl, R.M., Latner, J.D., O'Brien, K., et al. (2015). "Cross-National Perspectives About Weight-Based Bullying in Youth: Nature, Extent and Remedies." *Pediatric Obesity*, published online July 6, 2015.

125 Harris, R. (2008). *The Happiness Trap: How to Stop Struggling and Start Living*. Boston: Trumpeter.

Manson, M. (2012). "Your Two Minds." markmanson.net, December 7, 2012.

126 Mann, T., Tomiyama, A.J., Westling, E., et al. (2007). "Medicare's Search for Effective Obesity Treatments: Diets Are Not the Answer." *American Psychologist*, 62(3), 220–33.

127 Booth, J.N, Leary, S.D., Joinson, C., et al. (2013). "Associations Between Objectively Measured Physical Activity and Academic Attainment in Adolescents from a UK Cohort." *British Journal of Sports Medicine*, published online October 21, 2013.

128 Whiteman, H. (2013). "Aerobic Fitness Boosts Memory and Learning in Children." medicalnewstoday.com, September 12, 2013.

129 Sibley, B.A., and Etnier, J.L. (2003). "The Relationship Between Physical Activity and Cognition in Children: A Meta-Analysis." *Pediatric Exercise Science*, 15, 243–56.

130 Martikainen, S., Pesonen, A.K., Lahti, J., et al. (2013). "Higher Levels of Physical Activity Are Associated with Lower Hypothalamic-Pituitary-Adrenocortical Axis Reactivity to Psychosocial Stress in Children." *Journal of Clinical Endocrinology and Metabolism*, 98(4), E619–27.

131 WebMD (2014). "Exercise and Depression." webmd.com.

132 Baker, C.W., and Brownell, K.D. (2000). "Physical Activity and Maintenance of Weight Loss: Physiological and Psychological Mechanisms." In Bouchard, C., ed., *Physical Activity and Obesity*, Champaign, IL: Human Kinetics, pp. 311–28.

133 Bailey, D.A., Mckay, H.A, Mirwald, R.L., et al. (1999). "A Six-Year Longitudinal Study of the Relationship of Physical Activity to Bone Mineral Accrual in Growing Children: The University of Saskatchewan Bone Mineral Accrual Study." *Journal of Bone Mineral Research*, 14(10), 1672–79.

134 Centers for Disease Control and Prevention. "Physical Activity and Health: The Benefits of Physical Activity." cdc.gov.

135 Centers for Disease Control and Prevention. "How Much Physical Activity Do Children Need?" cdc.gov.

US Department of Health and Human Services (2008). *2008 Physical Activity Guidelines for Americans.* Washington, DC: US Department of Health and Human Services. health .gov/PAguidelines/guidelines/default.aspx.

136 Centers for Disease Control and Prevention (2014). "Youth Risk Behavior Surveillance – United States, 2013." *Morbidity and Mortatlity Weekly Report (MMWR)*, 63(4).

137 National Physical Activity Plan Alliance (2014). *The 2014 United States Report Card on Physical Activity for Children and Youth.* Columbia SC: National Physical Activity Plan. physicalactivityplan.org.

138 Sallis, J.F. (2014). "Influences on Physical Activity of Children, Adolescents, and Adults." *PCPFC Research Digest*, 1(7). presidentschallenge.org/informed/digest/docs/199408digest.pdf.

139 McKenzie, T.L., Sallis, J.F, Nader, P.R., et al. (1992). "Anglo and Mexican-American Preschoolers at Home and at Recess: Activity Patterns and Environmental Influences." *Journal of Developmental and Behavioral Pediatrics*, 13(3), 173–80.

140 Stucky-Ropp, R.C., and DiLorenzo, T.M. (1993). "Determinants of Exercise in Children." *Preventive Medicine*, 22, 880–89.

141 Epstein, L.H., Smith, J.A., Vara, L.S., and Rodefer, J.S. (1991). "Behavioral Economic Analysis of Activity Choice in Obese Children." *Health Psychology*, 10(5), 311–16.

142 Dishman, R.K., Sallis, J.F., and Orenstein, D.R. (1994). "Determinants and Interventions for Physical Activity and Exercise." In C. Bouchard, R.J. Shephard, and T. Stephens (Eds.), *Physical Activity, Fitness, and Health: International Proceedings and Consensus Statement*, Champaign, IL: Human Kinetics Publishers, pp. 214–38.

143 Sallis, J.F., Prochaska, J.J., and Taylor, W.C. (2000). "A Review of Correlates of Physical Activity of Children and Adolescents." *Medicine and Science in Sports and Exercise*, 32(5), 963–75.

144 American Heart Association (2013). "Children's Cardiovascular Fitness Declining Worldwide." American Heart Association Meeting Report: Abstract 13498, November 19, 2013.

Paddock, C. (2013). "Children Less Fit Than Their Parents." medicalnewstoday.com, November 19, 2013.

145 Ibid.

146 National Association for Sport and Physical Education and American Heart Association (2012). *2012 Shape of the Nation Report: Status of Physical Education in the USA*. Reston, VA: American Alliance for Health, Physical Education, Recreation and Dance.

147 McCullick, B.A., Baker, T., Tomporowski, P.D., et al. (2012). "An Analysis of State Physical Education Policies." *Journal of Teaching in Physical Education*, 31(2), 200–210.

148 Strauss, V. (2014). "Why So Many Kids Can't Sit Still in School Today." *Washington Post*, July 8, 2014.

Strauss, V. (2014). "A Therapist Goes to Middle School and Tries to Sit Still and Focus. She Can't. Neither Can the Kids." *Washington Post*, December 13, 2014.

149 McCullick, Baker, and Tomporowski, "An Analysis of State Physical Education Policies."

150 New York State. "Part 135: Health, Physical Education and Recreation." In *Official Compilation of Codes, Rules and Regulations of the State of New York*. p12.nysed.gov/ciai/pe/pub/part135.pdf. See Regulation 11.135.4(c)(2)(a).

151 Council on Sports Medicine and Fitness and Council on School Health. (2006). "Active Healthy Living: Prevention of Childhood Obesity Through Increased Physical Activity." Policy statement. *Pediatrics*, 117, 1834.

152 Sallis, J.F., Alcaraz, J.E., McKenzie, T.L., et al. (1992). "Parental Behavior in Relation to Physical Activity and Fitness in 9-Year-Old Children." *American Journal of Diseases of Children*, 146(11), 1383–88.

Sallis, J.F., and Hovell, M.F. (1990). "Determinants of Exercise Behavior." *Exercise and Sports Sciences Reviews*, 18, 307–30.

153 Matz, J. (2015). "Common Mistakes Parents Make About Their Kid's Weight." http://thebodyisnotanapology.com/magazine/9-common-mistakes-parents-make-about-their-kids-weight/

CHAPTER 10

154 Verheijden, M.W., Bakx, J.C., van Weel, C, et al. (2005). "Role of Social Support in Lifestyle-Focused Weight Management Interventions." *European Journal of Clinical Nutrition*, 59, Suppl 1, S179–86.

Reblin, M., and Uchino, B.N. (2008). "Social and Emotional Support and Its Implications for Health." *Current Opinion in Psychiatry*, 21(2), 201–5.

155 Hunter-Geboy, C. (1995). "Assertiveness Techniques: A Lesson Plan from *Life Planning Education: A Youth Development Program (Chapter 3)*." advocatesforyouth.org.

Women's and Children's Health Network. "Assertiveness – What It Means." cyh.com.

156 Lyness, D. (2014). "Asking for Help: Getting Past Obstacles." teenshealth.org.

157 Center for Nutrition Policy and Promotion. (1995). *The Healthy Eating Index*. Washington, DC: US Department of Agriculture.

158 Fox, M.K., Gordon, A., Nogales, R., and Wilson, A. (2009). "Availability and Consumption of Competitive Foods in US Public Schools." *Journal of the American Dietetic Association*, 109(2 Suppl), S57–66.

159 See 210.11 of the NSLP regulations and Section 220.12 of the SBP regulations. fns.usda.gov/sites/default/files/7cfr210_13_1.pdf.

160 US Department of Agriculture. "Healthier School Day: Tools for Schools: Focusing on Smart Snacks." fns.usda.gov/healthierschoolday/tools-schools-smart-snacks.

US Department of Agriculture. "Smart Snacks in School: USDA's 'All Foods Sold in Schools' Standards." fns.usda.gov/sites/default/files/allfoods_flyer.pdf.

161 US Department of Agriculture. (2013). "USDA Proposes Standards to Provide Healthy Food Options in Schools." Release No. 0019.13, February 1, 2013. fns.usda.gov/pressrelease/2013/001913.

162 Office of Disease Prevention and Health Promotion, US Department of Health and Human Services. (2015). "Part D. Chapter 6: Cross-Cutting Topics of Health Importance." In *Scientific Report of the 2015 Dietary Guidelines Advisory Committee*. health.gov/dietaryguidelines/2015-scientific-report.

163 Goodman, E. (1999). "Ads Pollute Most Everything in Sight." *Albuquerque Journal*, June 27, 1999. C3.

164 McNeal, J. (1992). *Kids as Customers: A Handbook of Marketing to Children*. Lexington, MA: Lexington Books.

165 Tavernise, S. (2015). "Obesity Rises Despite All Efforts to Fight It, U.S. Health Officials Say." *The New York Times*, November 12, 2015.

Wang, D.D., Li, Y., Chiuve, S.E., et al. (2015). "Improvements in US Diet Helped Reduce Disease Burden and Lower Premature Deaths, 1999–2012; Overall Diet Remains Poor." *Health Affairs*, 34(11), 1916–22.

166 Cullen K.W., and Zakeri, L. (2004). "Fruits, Vegetables, Milk, and Sweetened Beverages Consumption and Access to à La Carte/Snack Bar Meals at School." *American Journal of Public Health*, 94(3), 463–67.

Cullen, K.W., Eagan, J., Baranowski, T., et al. (2000). "Effect of a La Carte and Snack Bar Foods at School on Children's Lunchtime Intake of Fruits and Vegetables." *Journal of the American Dietetic Association*, 100(12), 1482–86.

Dietz, W.H. (1993). "Childhood Obesity." In R.M. Suskind and L. Lewinter-Suskind, *Textbook of Pediatric Nutrition*, 2nd ed., New York: Raven Press, pp. 281–84.

Harnack L., Stang J., and Story, M. (1999). "Soft Drink Consumption Among US Children and Adolescents: Nutritional Consequences." *Journal of the American Dietetic Association*, 99(4), 436–41.

CHAPTER 11

167 Perri, M.G., Nezu, A.M, McKelvey, W.F., et al. (2001). "Relapse Prevention Training and Problem-Solving Therapy in the Long-term Management of Obesity." *Journal of Consulting and Clinical Psychology*, 69(4), 722–26.

168 Corsica, J., Hood, M.M., Katterman, S., et al. (2014). "Development of a Novel Mindfulness and Cognitive Behavioral Intervention for Stress Eating: A Comparative Pilot Study." *Eating Behaviors*, 15(4), 694–99.

Courbasson, C.M., Nishikawa, Y., and Shapira, L.B. (2011). "Mindfulness-Action Based Cognitive Behavioral Therapy for Concurrent Binge Eating Disorder and Substance Use Disorders." *Eating Disorders*, 19(1), 17–33.

169 Riccardo, D.G., Calugi, S., and El Ghoch, M. (2015). "Increasing Adherence to Diet and Exercise Through Cognitive Behavioural Strategies." In A. Lenzi, S. Migliaccio, and L.M. Donini (Eds.), *Multidisciplinary Approach to Obesity: From Assessment to Treatment*. Cham, Switzerland: Springer International Publishing, pp. 327–35.

Mariani, S., Watanabe, M., Lubrano, C., et al. (2015). "Interdisciplinary Approach to Obesity." In Lenzi, Migliaccio, and Donini, *Multidisciplinary Approach to Obesity*, pp. 337–42.

170 Forman, E.M., Hoffman, K.L., McGrath, K.B., et al. (2007). "A Comparison of Acceptance- and Control-Based Strategies for Coping with Food Cravings: An Analog Study." *Behaviour Research and Therapy*, 45(10), 2372–86.

Lillis, J., Hayes, S.C., Bunting, K., and Masuda, A. (2009). "Teaching Acceptance and Mindfulness to Improve the Lives of the Obese: A Preliminary Test of a Theoretical Model." *Annals of Behavioral Medicine*, 37(1), 58–69.

Sairanen, E., Lappalainen, R., Lapveteläinen, A., et al. (2014). "Flexibility in Weight Management." *Eating Behaviors*, 15(2), 218–24.

RESOURCES

NUTRITION INFORMATION

Nutrition and the Health of Young People –
   Centers for Disease Control and Prevention
   cdc.gov/healthyschools/nutrition/facts.htm

Child Nutrition – National Institutes of Health
   nlm.nih.gov/medlineplus/childnutrition.html

Child Nutrition – US Department of Agriculture
   http://fnic.nal.usda.gov/lifecycle-nutrition/child-nutrition

Choose My Plate – US Department of Agriculture
   choosemyplate.gov/children-over-five.html

Dietary Guidelines – US Department of Agriculture
   cnpp.usda.gov/dietaryguidelines

Go!Healthy Kids Health and Nutrition – The Children's Aid Society
   childrensaidsociety.org/kids-health-nutrition

The Healthy Eating Index – US Department of Agriculture
   cnpp.usda.gov/sites/default/files/healthy_eating_index/HEI89-90report.pdf

KidsHealth
   http://kidshealth.org/parent/centers/fitness_nutrition_center.html

Preteens and Teenagers – US Department of Agriculture
   http://fnic.nal.usda.gov/consumers/ages-stages/preteens-teenagers

Take Charge of Your Health: A Guide for Teenagers –
   National Institutes of Health
   http://win.niddk.nih.gov/publications/pdfs/teenblackwhite3.pdf

Teen Nutrition – US Department of Agriculture
   http://fnic.nal.usda.gov/lifecycle-nutrition/teen-nutrition

We Can! Ways to Enhance Children's Activity and Nutrition – National Institute
   of Health and US Department of Health and Human Service
   nhlbi.nih.gov/health/educational/wecan

Health Conscious Eating: Kids Recipes: Healthy Cookbook for Beginners by Health Conscious Eating

The Truly Healthy Family Cookbook: Mega-nutritious Meals That Are Inspired, Delicious and Fad-Free by Tina Ruggiero

Meal Simple: The Camp Shane Cookbook. Quick, Easy, Delicious and Healthy Recipes by Camp Shane and Shane Diet and Fitness Resorts

Little Bites: 100 Healthy, Kid-Friendly Snacks by Christine Chitnis and Sarah Waldman

The America's Test Kitchen Healthy Family Cookbook: A New, Healthier Way to Cook Everything from America's Most Trusted Test Kitchen by America's Test Kitchen

Healthy Recipes: A Toolkit for Healthy Teens and Strong Families by US Department of Health and Human Services

Healthy Start Kids' Cookbook: Fun and Healthful Recipes That Kids Can Make Themselves by Sandra K. Nissenberg

Best Lunch Box Ever: Ideas and Recipes for School Lunches Kids Will Love by Katie Sullivan Morford (author) and Jennifer Martiné (photographer)

101 Recipes for a Healthy Kids Diet: A Parents Guide to Healthy Snacks, Sack Lunches, and Desserts That Your Kids Will Love by Minute Help Guides

44 Things Parents Should Know About Healthy Cooking for Kids by Rock Harper

Smart School Time Recipes: The Breakfast, Snack, and Lunchbox Cookbook for Healthy Kids and Adults by Alisa Fleming

Healthy Juices for Healthy Kids: Over 70 Juice and Smoothie Recipes for Kids of All Ages by Wendy Sweetser

Overweight Kids in a Toothpick World by Brenda Wollenberg, BSW, RHN

NUTRITION AND HEALTHY EATING APPS

Awesome Eats – Whole Kids Foundation

Cooking Light magazine – Time Inc.

Figure Facts Teen Nutrition – Figure Facts LLC

Girl Zone Challenge – Girl Zone Corp.

LaLa Lunch Box – LaLa Lunchbox, LLC

Meal Makeovers – Mobile Skillet, LLC

Peekaboo Fridge – Night & Day Studios, Inc.

FITNESS RESOURCES

Exercise, Fitness, and Nutrition for Teens
http://kids.usa.gov/teens/exercise-fitness-nutrition

Find Walking Tracks, Parks, and Locations
fitlink.com/walking-tracks-parks

Fitness for Kids Who Don't Like Sports – KidsHealth
http://kidshealth.org/parent/nutrition_center/staying_fit/hate_sports.html

Getting Fit Interactively – kidnetic.com

Motivating Kids to Get Fit – PBS Kids
pbs.org/parents/food-and-fitness/sport-and-fitness/motivating-kids-to-get-fit

Physical Activity Guidelines for Americans – The Office of Disease Prevention
and Health Promotion (ODPHP), US Department of Health and Human
Services (HHS)
health.gov/paguidelines

FITNESS VIDEO GAMES

Wii Shaun White Snowboarding

Wii Walk It Out

Wii Zumba Kids

Wii Just Dance

Wii Nickelodeon Fit

Wii Fit

Wii Fit Plus

Xbox 360 Just Dance Kids

Xbox 360 Zumba Fitness

Xbox 360 Shape Up

PS3 Zumba Fitness

PS3 Just Dance

PS3 EA Sports Active 2

FITNESS APPS

FitQuest Lite – JogHop

Girl Zone Challenge – Girl Zone Corp.

Kids Yogaverse: I Am Sun, I Am Moon – Gramercy Consultants

iBitz by Geopalz: Kids – GeoPalz LLC

Iron Kids – American Academy of Pediatrics

Yoga by Teens – Let It Go Yoga

Youth Fitness Free – Boyan Dzhambazov

Youth Fitness Pro - Boyan Dzhambazov

Super Stretch Yoga (also in Spanish) – Health & Fitness

MINDFULNESS APPS

Insight Timer – Bradley Fullmer

Sitting Still – MindApps

Smiling Mind

SoulBuddy EN – Sophie Loof Martensson

Stop, Breathe and Think – Tools for Peace

Take a Chill – Stressed Teens – Channel Capital, LLC

ZenFriend – Meditation Timer and Guided Meditations – Small-n-Tall

ADVOCACY

Healthy Kids, Healthy Communities – Robert Wood Johnson Foundation
healthykidshealthycommunities.org

Let's Move! – Launched by Michelle Obama
letsmove.gov

Obesity Action Coalition
obesityaction.org

University of Connecticut Rudd Center for Food Policy and Obesity
uconnruddcenter.org

ACKNOWLEDGMENTS

DEEP GRATITUDE GOES TO my loving and gracious husband, Eric, and our children, Addison, Foster, Wyatt, and Cora. This book is a product of their everlasting patience, love, and support.

And also to the committed and skilled individuals at The Experiment for their support: Matthew Lore, Dan O'Connor, Jennifer Hergenroeder, Vivienne Woodward, Jeanne Tao, Sarah Smith, and Sarah Schneider. To my editor at The Experiment, Allie Bochicchio, I greatly appreciate all your guidance and vision. Thank you to Katie McHugh Malm for your editorial support. To Molly Cavanaugh, a former editor at The Experiment, who pitched and helped construct the book, I appreciate your belief in me and for helping to get the message out to the public.

Thank you to Don Fehr, my literary agent at Trident Media Group. I appreciate your taking a chance on me and for "getting" my passion for the work I do and the mission of this book.

I am thankful for Julie Mosow's editorial guidance. I greatly appreciate the endless hours my father, Steven Farkas, spent reading and rereading my material, from the outset through to the finished product.

I am indebted to the staff members and the kids and teens at the Boys & Girls Club in Mount Vernon, New York. A special thank-you to Mel Campos, chief professional officer, and Ms. Halima Penny, teen coordinator at the club. I was fortunate to meet and interact with incredible kids and parents during my focus groups, and they were generous with their time and so forthcoming.

Deep gratitude goes to David Ettenberg and Ziporah Janowski, the directors at Camp Shane and Shane Fitness and Diet Resorts, for the opportunity to create the CBT program at their sites for their staff, coaches, and campers, who continue to motivate me through their dedication, kindness, and openness.

Thank you to my peer readers who offered their skill and guidance: Dr. Eve Goldstein, Dr. Heather Maguire, Lori Ginsberg, Caroline Martin, and Alison Kaslow. Thank you, as well, to the knowledgeable and talented group of nutritionists, nurse practitioners, and health coaches who comprised my professional focus groups: Wendy Sterling, Kirsti Pesso, Sue Adams, Lisa Ellis, Ilanit Blumenfeld, Tamra Rosenfeld, Jennifer McGurk, and Elyse Falk.

I especially want to thank Dr. Aaron T. Beck, Dr. Judith S. Beck, Dr. Marci G. Fox, Dr. Steven C. Hayes, Dr. John P. Forsyth, Dr. Georg H. Eifert, Dr. Russ Harris, Pema Chödrön, and Dr. Margaret Gibelman, all of whom I had the benefit of personally learning from and who have greatly informed my writing as well as facilitated growth in both my professional and personal life. Finally, I want to thank my patients, students, friends, and colleagues who continue to inspire me. I have the benefit of learning something new every day, which I'm eternally grateful for and which profoundly influences my writing, my practice, and my life.

INDEX

Gaesser, Glenn, 145
glucose. *See* sugar
goals. *See* health goals and needs
governmental nutrition programs, 198–202
gratitude, encouraging, 97, 166–67, 218–19, 222, 225–28
grocery shopping, 127
growth spurts, 71, 123, 152
guided imagery, 19, 62, 217
guilt. *See* shame and guilt

HALT, 66, 67
happiness, focus on, 21–22
Harris, Russ, 22
Hayes, Steven, 10
health, defined, 35
health costs, 36
healthful behaviors
    advertising and marketing, influence of, 157, 199
    advocating, 6–9
    assessing current, 44–45
    commitment to, 4, 110, 205, 211
    80/20 rule, 145, 213
    evaluating, 52–56
    family's influence on, 75–76, 112–13
    friendships, influence on, 150–52
    HALT strategy for, 66, 67
    importance of, communicating, 139–41
    instant gratification feelings, 156–57
    intuitive eating practices, 70–75
    knowledge base on, 144–47, 148–49
    modeling of by parents and family, 113–15
    moderation in eating, 70, 123–24, 145–47, 213
    personal importance of, 38–41
    serving sizes, 70–73, 127, 194, 197, 200
    SMART goals, 126, 157
    thought processing, 12–16
    value-based behaviors, barriers to, 35, 45, 49, 172–78
    value-based behaviors, evaluating, 31–32, 39, 41–47, 65
health goals and needs
    asserting and expressing, 188–95
    for fitness and physical activity, 169
    giving in to cravings *vs.* sabotaging, 65
    health-based values, 4, 47–48, 110, 205, 211
    health-based values *vs.*, 33–35
    healthful behaviors, 44–45
    open dialogue about, 145–47
    self-efficacy for, 116–19, 130, 170
    SMART goals, 126, 157
    teamwork in families for, 125–28, 139
    See also challenges, overcoming
Healthy, Hunger-Free Kids Act of 2010, 198
helplessness, feelings of, 116–19
hiding food, 122–25
high-fat diets, research on, 146–47
high-sugar diets, research on, 146–47
hormones
    developmental changes and, 39, 139, 150–55, 176
    leptin, 73, 146
    stress hormones, 19
How to Get Your Kid to Eat, But Not Too Much (Satter), 123

hunger
    binge eating, 56, 81, 108, 137, 145–46
    connecting to feelings of, 156–57
    desire *vs.*, 63
    emotional *vs.* physical hunger, 66–68
    evaluating self for, 54
    instant gratification feelings and, 156–57
    rating hunger, 59
    thirst *vs.*, 57, 58
    types of, differentiating, 56–59, 70
hunger scale, 56–57
hyper-palatable foods, 146
hypocrisy, 113

identity. *See* self-awareness; self-identity
imagery exercises, 19, 62, 217
immune system
    fitness and physical activity, 170
    mindfulness, impact on, 19
imperfections, accepting, 47, 51, 135, 191, 204–5, 213
implicit messages, 135–36
impulsive behavior, 71, 78, 115, 144
    developmental changes and, 153
    parents challenged by, 135
    stereotypes about, 115, 133, 135, 156
    thought processing, 14–16
impulsive eating, 60, 62, 67, 71, 78, 105, 117, 204
independence and freedom
    core values on, 31–32, 40
    cost of being overweight to, 37–38, 49, 50
Instagram, 155–56
instant gratification, 156–57
Institute of Medicine, 198
insulin, 146
integrity, as core value, 31
intuition, noticing, 101, 102
intuitive eating practices, 70–75
isolation and loneliness, 7, 134, 150, 155, 160–61
    emotional eating and, 65–66

Jakubczak, Jane, 67–68
Johnson, Carol, 145
journaling, 55–56
Journal of the American Medical Association, 1
judgment. *See* criticism and judgment
junk food, label of, 27, 124, 134, 159
justification, 84

Kabat-Zinn, Jon, 18
knowledge base, 144–47, 148–49

labeling and name-calling, 43, 122, 137–38, 156
labeling foods, 27, 124, 126–28, 134, 137, 159
language and terminology
    body language, 28, 111, 135–39, 190, 192
    empowering terminology, 138
    frame of reference and language, 27–28
    negative expressions, 122
    nonjudgmental language, 136–37
    thoughts and feelings, impact on, 27–28
laxatives, 7, 153

leftovers
    candy and unhealthy snacks, 197
    cravings and, 12, 60, 194
    eating out and, 193, 194
    serving size and, 73
leptin, 73, 146
life expectancies, 120, 170
Like Mother, Like Daughter (Waterhouse), 115
listening, active, 6, 85, 120–25, 131–32, 138–39, 162
loneliness. *See* isolation and loneliness
lovability, feelings of, 116–19
    See also self-acceptance and self-love

magazines, cultural influence of, 157, 159, 199
magnification and minimization, 82
Mann, Traci, 107
marketing, food and beverage, 157, 158–9, 199
Mazlish, Elaine, 142
meal replacements, 107–8
media and technology
    advertising and marketing, 157, 199
    apps, mindfulness, 19–20
    cultural influence of, 155–60
    instant gratification and, 156–57
    magazines, 157, 159, 199
    screen time and weight gain, 2–3, 128
    social media, 2–3, 155–56, 158
    thinness, idealization of, 35, 139, 155–58
meditation, benefits of, 19–20
mental filters, 82
metabolism
    aging and changes in, 9
    dieting and decrease in, 108
    differences in, 9, 71, 116, 146
    eating behaviors, effect on, 108, 146
    for kids and teens *vs.* adults, 71
    physical activity and, 146, 170
micromanaging behavior, 70, 71, 121, 129
mindfulness
    apps for, 19
    balanced thinking, 87–92, 102–4, 183
    benefits of, 2–4, 11, 19–21
    committed action, 11, 26, 49, 52
    defined, 18
    happiness *vs.*, 21–22
    healthful eating *vs.* dieting, 70–75
    intuitive eating practices, 70–75
    language and frame of reference, 27–28
    listening to thoughts and feelings, 13–14
    meditation, benefits of, 19–20
    practicing, 20–21
    present moment, 18–21, 25–26, 28–29
    reframing thoughts, 17, 18, 26–27, 92, 102,
        165–67, 183, 206
    space between feelings and action, 25–26, 28–29
    thought patterns, understanding, 16–18
    thought processing, 10–16
    thoughts and feelings, accepting and
        understanding, 16–18, 21–26
    visualization, 19, 27–28
mindfulness-based activities, 2–4, 11, 18–21, 62, 63,
    115, 217
mind games, 10–16
mindless eating. *See* impulsive eating

mind over muffin, 26–27
mind reading, 83
minimization and magnification, 82
mirroring, 113–15, 134, 139, 141
moderation in eating, 70, 123–24, 145–47, 213
motivation
    criticism and stinking thinking, 80–85, 126
    fitness and physical activity, 168–69, 178–80
    health values, 30, 32–33
    increasing and supporting, 6–9
    practicing (4Ps) for, 64–65, 108–9
    stereotypes and labels, 43, 122, 137–38, 156
    value-based behaviors, 31, 43–47
motivational interviewing (MI), 6
muscle strength, 44, 109, 146, 170–71, 175

name-calling and labeling, 43, 122, 137–38, 156
National Association of Sports and Physical
    Education (NASPE), 175
National Health and Nutrition Examination Survey,
    147
National Physical Activity Plan Alliance, 171–72
National School Lunch Program (NSLP), 198, 200–1
National Sleep Foundation, 128
neurochemical rewards for food, 3, 73, 74, 146, 204
nutrition
    books on, 5
    knowledge base on, 144–47, 148–49
    public education campaigns on, 2, 199–200
    school-based programs for, 198–202
nutritionists, 84, 118, 145, 147

obesity
    advertising and marketing, 157, 199
    causes of, 145–47
    cost of, 36–38, 49, 50
    as disease, 145
    future health concerns and, 134–35
    high-fat diets, 146
    physiological reasons for, 146–47
    poverty and, 199–200
    screen time and weight gain, 2–3, 128
    stereotypes about, 156
    in United States, 1–2
observations *vs.* judgments, 164–66
open dialogue, creating, 6–9, 133–39, 145–49
open-ended questions, 6, 85, 124, 138
overeating. *See* unhealthful behaviors
overweight people
    cost of weight gain, 36–38, 49, 50
    physical and psychological effects for, 1
    screen time and weight gain, 2–3, 128
    in United States, 1–2
    See also obesity; weight biases and discrimination;
        weight gain

parental modeling, 2, 113–15, 120–22, 137–39,
    172–73
parents
    bullying, reactions to, 161
    communication, 2, 6–9, 115, 133–36
    cultural influences on, 159–60
    health-based values of, 16–18, 31

FREE YOUR CHILD FROM OVEREATING

INDEX

ABOUT THE AUTHOR

MICHELLE P. MAIDENBERG, PhD, MPH, LCSW-R, is the president and clinical director of Westchester Group Works, a center for group therapy, and also maintains a private practice serving individuals, couples, and families. She created and coordinates the Cognitive-Behavioral Therapy program at Camp Shane, a health and weight-management camp for kids and teens in Arizona, California, Georgia, New York, and Texas, and Shane Diet and Fitness Resorts for young adults and adults in New York. Dr. Maidenberg is cofounder and clinical director of Thru My Eyes, a nonprofit that allows individuals with life-threatening diseases to leave clinically guided video legacies for their loved ones. She teaches at New York University in their graduate program in the Silver School of Social Work. Dr. Maidenberg is a consultant and trainer and often presents at conferences and publishes on the topics of health and wellness, parenting, mindfulness, socialization, anxiety, trauma, assertiveness training, and group treatment. She has contributed to articles in *The New York Times*, *Fitness*, *Shape*, *Parents*, *Parenting*, and more.